£2·99.
pb

Epidemiology

Epidemiology

[An introductory
text for medical
and other
health science
students]

Second Edition

David Christie
MD, FRACP, FAFOM
University of Newcastle

Ian Gordon
MSc, PhD
University of Melbourne

Richard Heller
MD, FRCP, FRACP,
FFPHM, FAFPHM
University of Newcastle

UNSW
PRESS

Published by
UNIVERSITY OF NEW SOUTH WALES PRESS LTD
Sydney 2052
Telephone (02) 9398 8900   Fax (02) 9398 3408

© D. Christie, I. Gordon, R. Heller
Second edition published in 1997
First edition published in 1987
First edition reprinted with minor amendments 1990, 1994

National Library of Australia
Cataloguing-in-Publication entry:

Christie, David, 1935- .
Epidemiology, an introductory text for medical and other
health science students.

2nd ed.
Bibliography.
Includes index.
ISBN 0 86840 400 4

1. Epidemiology. I. Gordon, Ian, 1956- . II. Heller, Richard F.
III. Title.

614.4

Design: Mango Design Group
Managing Editor: Nada Madjar
Printer: Ligare, Riverwood, NSW
Production Manager: Di Quick
Publisher: John Elliot

CONTENTS

FOREWORD
TO THE
FIRST EDITION

'NEXT PATIENT, PLEASE!'—and then we do our best to diagnose and treat whoever walks in. The consultation is the central activity of medicine, and for some doctors it is the whole of medicine: they never take off their clinical blinkers. What this book does is indicate how a wider outlook can get better results—better use of our limited medical resources, a reduction in the burden of end-stage incurable disease, and it is intellectually more interesting and professionally more satisfying.

'Why did this patient fall ill now with this disease? How might the illness have been prevented? How many more people are there, out there in the community, with the same condition, undiagnosed? Would screening help? How efficient is the diagnostic process anyway? And can we believe the remarkable therapeutic claims of the glossy advertisements? What really happens to our patients in the long-term?'

Questions such as these extend the horizon of thinking. They make the practice of medicine more interesting, and they help us to move out of the purely passive 'next patient, please!' mode into a more informed and critical mode of thinking. They are the starting point for medical planning, setting priorities and making better use of our efforts and resources.

These questions are epidemiological. They should be an integral part of every doctor's thinking, but to frame them clearly and to get the right answers calls for specific skills and understanding. This book provides them, and it does so in a clear, no-nonsense, readable way. It will help its readers to be more complete doctors.

Geoffrey Rose DM, DSc, FRCP, FFCM
Division of Medical Statistics and Epidemiology
London School of Hygiene and Tropical Medicine

Professor Rose died on 12 November 1993. His obituary, by David Barker, concluded with the following words:

Geoffrey Rose's public and research career was marked by wisdom, wit and generosity, and was guided by his profound religious beliefs. He set us an example.

(Brit. Med. J. 307: 1418 (1993))

PREFACE

The second edition, like the first, is intended as an undergraduate text, introducing population-based research to students in medicine and the health sciences. It has been extensively rewritten, with updating of relevant vital statistics and the addition of a new chapter on diagnostic tests and screening for diseases. Except for a few instances where important principles are brought out, all references have been updated, using mainly Australian works. The chapter on the randomised controlled trial in particular has been modified to emphasise the use of this technique in research problems, which may be of more interest to non-medical students. Thus the discussion on ethics in this context has been expanded.

The practice of including questions at the end of each chapter has been continued in this edition, but in response to many requests from our own students we have added model answers. Since we regard the questions and their answers to be integral parts of the learning process, both have been inserted at the end of relevant chapters.

The parts of the book related to statistics have been modified by removing the artificial Part I and Part II Divisions. Some of the more technical material on distribution theory, in particular integrals and summations used in the definitions of expectations and variances, have been deleted. In the second edition a greater emphasis is put on the normal distribution, since it is the basis of many of the confidence intervals given, and the students will use it extensively should they choose to go further in statistics or population research. In Chapter 13, a table of sample sizes for comparing two proportions has been added.

In general, this second edition reflects almost ten years' further experience by the authors in teaching of and research in epidemiology and statistics. We trust it will be a helpful introduction to this expanding field.

David Christie

ACKNOWLEGEMENTS

The authors wish to express their appreciation to the following publishers who have kindly given their permission for the use of copyright material:

British Heart Journal, for the material used in Table 5.7

British Medical Journal, for material used in Tables 4.5, 4.7, 4.8 and 7.2

Medical Journal of Australia, for material used in Tables 5.2 and 5.4, and Figure 7.2

International Journal of Epidemiology, for material used in Figure 8.1

New England Journal of Medicine, for material used in Table 7.4

Oxford University Press for material used in Figure 7.5

Blackwell Science Pty Ltd for material used in Figure 2.7

ABBREVIATIONS

ABS	Australian Bureau of Statistics
AIDS	acquired immune deficiency syndrome
AZT	Zidovudine (an anti-retroviral drug active against HIV)
BP	blood pressure
CASS	Coronary Artery Surgery Study
CCU	Coronary Care Unit
CFR	case-fatality ratio
CHD	coronary heart disease
CI	confidence interval
CL	confidence limits
DRG	diagnostic related group
ECG	electrocardiogram
HIV	human immunodeficiency virus
ICD	International Classification of Diseases
IHD	ischaemic heart disease
IMR	infant mortality rate
IQ	intelligence quotient
JVP	jugular venous pressure
MI	myocardial infarction
MRC	Medical Research Council
MRI	magnetic resonance imaging
OR	odds ratio
pdf	probability density function
PHC	primary hepatocellular carcinoma
Pr	probability
PYR	person years at risk
RR	relative risk
RCT	randomised controlled trial
SMF	synthetic mineral fibres
SMR	standardised mortality ratio *or* standardised morbidity ratio

CHAPTER ONE
INTRODUCTION

Epidemiology may be formally defined as the study of the distribution and determinants of disease in human populations. Its purpose is to enable us to gain a greater understanding of the causation and natural history of disease and to develop and evaluate strategies in the prevention, diagnosis, and management of disease; it also helps us with the ordering of priorities of resource allocation in health care.

Clinicians study disease in individual patients, write up interesting and unusual case-reports, and note clusters of patients with the same rare disease. The association between occupationally determined exposure to vinyl chloride monomer and development of angiosarcoma of the liver was recognised by an astute clinician seeing a cluster of rare cases. Laboratory researchers carry out controlled experiments within which biological systems can be explored and components changed. The epidemiologist works with populations, not individuals, and by the very nature of things this research is usually observational. In spite of the limitations imposed by this, epidemiology is important because, ultimately, human disease needs to be studied in people rather than in animals. Whilst epidemiologists traditionally studied disease in population settings, there is increasing interest by clinicians in using the principles of epidemiology to gain greater knowledge of their patients in hospital settings.

An example of the value of collecting apparently simple observations is given in Table 1.1 where, for each of the years 1979 to 1988, the number of children, aged 0–14 years, admitted to public hospitals in Newcastle with a diagnosis of 'asthma' is shown.[1] In 1979 there were 298 children admitted and the first question that springs to mind is whether this represents 'a lot or a little'. Common sense tells us that if these were the numbers for Sydney then asthma would not be a major public health problem, whereas if they related to a small country town there would be every cause for concern. Only by calculating a rate, by dividing the number of cases by the size of the population from which those cases are drawn, can disease occurrence in different places with

Table 1.1 Admission rates, per 1 000, of children aged less than 15 years of age for asthma, in the NSW city of Newcastle, in each of the years 1979–1988.

Year	1979	1980	1981	1982	1983	1984	1985	1986	1987	1988
No.	298	311	288	319	382	358	340	341	370	499
Rate	4.43	4.63	4.28	4.75	5.68	5.33	5.06	5.07	5.51	7.43

different population sizes be compared. A rate requires a numerator (cases) accruing over a specific time interval and a population which has been at risk during the same period (denominator). Crucial to the calculation of rates, shown in the third row of Table 1.1, are not only appropriate definitions of cases and populations but also a time period during which the cases occurred. In the present instance these are annual rates and their increase over the ten year period is a matter of concern. Sometimes, as in the Newcastle population aged less than 15 years, there was little change in the denominator over the ten years but population size can change quite importantly.

CASES

In this example a 'case' has been defined as a person aged 0–14 who has been recorded by one of the public hospitals serving Newcastle as an admission with the diagnosis of 'asthma' during the appropriate calendar year. The validity, or accuracy of these statistics depends on their completeness, on the quality of the record systems of the hospitals concerned, and on the diagnostic ability of the doctors who make that diagnosis.

Health service questions may often be reasonably answered by such a case definition, that is 'if a doctor says it is asthma then it is asthma', but where our interest lies in more complex questions such as understanding the nature of a disease process, we would be better served by a more precise and objective definition. Such a definition depends on the disease being studied but might sometimes include a microbiological component or, in the case of epidemiological studies of cancer, a diagnosis backed by a biopsy or autopsy report.

POPULATION
·······

Populations may be defined in various ways, the simplest being a school class roll or the payroll of a factory. In the asthma example shown in Table 1.1, the population was defined as the number of children aged 0–14 years residing in the 28 contiguous postcodes which form the geographic area of Newcastle on census night or, more precisely, the intercensal estimate of that population. Often it is of interest to specify the population in different ways and in Figure 1.1 the asthma admission rates of three different age groups are shown for the calendar years at the beginning, middle, and end of the period. It is clear that asthma is far more common in the youngest age group and least common in the 10–14 group. Further, it is apparent that whilst the rise in admission rates is evident in all age groups, it is greatest in the children 0–4 years of age.

When rates have been carefully calculated in this way there is a fair basis for comparison. An astute clinician might have formed the impression that the number of children with asthma diagnoses had been increasing and a perusal of hospital records would have confirmed this impression. Nevertheless, only by determining the rates is it possible to be certain of a trend over time and in certain circumstances, as where some change is relatively small but clinically important, such calculations may be the only way that such change comes to attention.

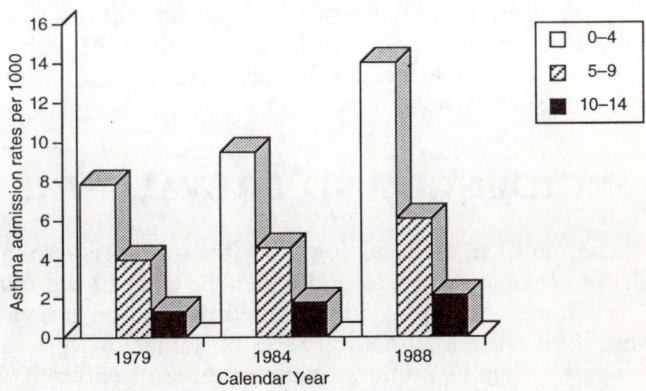

Figure 1.1 *Admission rates per 1 000 for asthma in three age groups in each of three selected years.*[1]

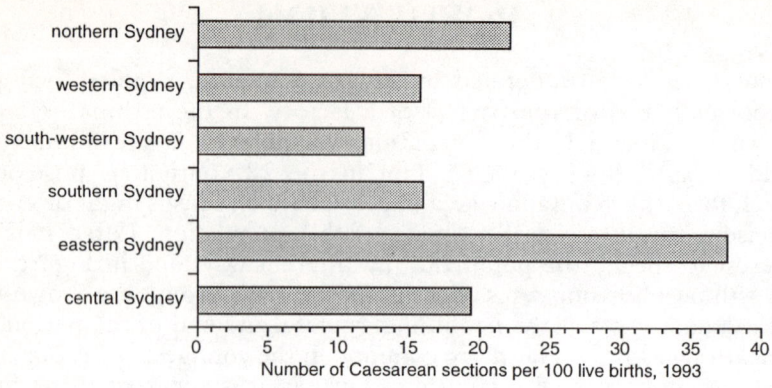

Figure 1.2 *Caesarean sections per 100 live births in six Sydney health areas, 1993.*

There are other ways of defining populations in special cases, such as the infant mortality rate where the denominator is the number of live births in the time period (or sometimes the total number of births). In Figure 1.2 the Caesarean section rates are shown for six metropolitan health areas of Sydney[2] and the denominator is the total number of live births (the sum of live births by vagina and by Caesarean section) in the same area and year. The marked variation between different geographic areas of Australia in the proportion of babies born by surgical intervention is well known and is thought to reflect, not anatomical differences in women living in different parts of the country, but rather the different beliefs held by the women and, perhaps more importantly, by their doctors.

INCIDENCE AND PREVALENCE

In the first chapter of an epidemiology text it is appropriate to introduce two words: *incidence* and *prevalence*. Incidence refers to the number of specified new events occurring in a defined population over a specific time period. The asthma admission rates in Table 1.1 were incidence rates because they had as numerator the number of children admitted to hospital with a specified condition from a defined population over a 12-month period. If instead of asthma the table had referred to the number of appendectomies that had been reported from the area over the time period, then that would also have been a rate.

Prevalence refers to the number of cases of disease that exist, in a defined population, at some point in time. If, during the first lecture on a Monday morning, we asked all students with a cold to put up their hands, then the point prevalence of the common cold might be:

Point prevalence: 10/180 = 55.6 per 1 000.
In a class of 180, 10 students on that Monday morning had a cold.

A statement like this is known as 'point prevalence' and is a very useful measure of long-standing chronic diseases. For short-lived ailments like the common cold, a more useful measure is 'period prevalence'; here we would ask the class members to put up their hands if at any time during the last month they had experienced a cold.

Period prevalence: 62/180 = 344.4 per 1 000 per month.

Incidence and prevalence are related through the duration of the illness. The prevalence of patients hospitalised with mental illness in Australia has fallen dramatically over the last 20 years; this is due more to a major shortening of the duration of hospitalisation regarded as appropriate for a psychotic episode than to a reduction in the incidence of the condition.

Cumulative Incidence

In a government department of 30 workers, all of whom were well at the beginning of the year, five had sick absences during the succeeding 12 months. The denominator of the sickness absence cumulative incidence is 30 and the numerator 5. Consequently the cumulative incidence of sickness absence is 5/30 (or 16.7 per 100) and describes the proportion of members of the department taking sickness absence leave during the last 12 months.

Incidence

In a seven bed nursing home unit over a period of five years, the beds were occupied by eight old people, each of whose stay is shown diagrammatically in Figure 1.3.

Three patients were discharged, one of them being readmitted at the beginning of 1994. Three patients died in the nursing home and another three were alive and in residence at the end of 1996.

If we wished to calculate the rate at which people die in the nursing home, the numerator is obviously three (the number of people who died) but what can we use as the denominator? Before we think of how this might be done, let us consider a new term, namely person years at risk.

50 people observed for a year   = 50 person years at risk
10 people observed for 5 years = 50 person years at risk
5 people observed for 10 years = 50 person years at risk

In Figure 1.3 the solid lines represent the time spent in the home by each of eight old people between 1992 and 1996. The total number of years spent in the home by the eight patients (that is when they were at risk of dying in the home) is 23. Thus the appropriate denominator is 23 person years and the death rate is 3/23 or 13 deaths per 100 person years. Incidence calculated in this manner, using person years, is also known as incidence density.

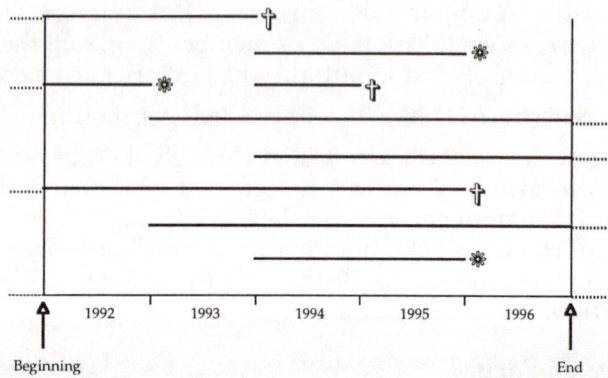

Figure 1.3 *A nursing home had seven beds and over the years 1992 to 1996 these were occupied by eight individuals. Each horizontal line represents a patient;* † *a death;* ✽ *a discharge from the nursing home.*

EXERCISES

Exercise 1.1
In Figure 1.2 the obstetric practices in different parts of Sydney were compared by the proportion of births that were delivered by Caesarean section in the relevant health areas. Can you think of a different denominator that could have been used in the comparison?

Exercise 1.2a
One of the more appalling military practices of the 1914–18 war was the use of mustard gas on the battlefield. Case[3] comments 'It was first used on the night of 17–18 July and after that date was used so extensively that areas of the (French) countryside became saturated with it and had to be abandoned by both sides'. The number of British cases of gas poisoning is recorded as being 160 970 and in 1930 there were 1 267 men who, on 1 January of that year, were alive and in receipt of a war pension for 'mustard gas poisoning'. Since these men were all on a pension, following them up until the end of 1952 was quite feasible and the number who had died, together with their date of death, was ascertained by Case. The deaths from any cause and

those from lung cancer were compared with those expected of the general British population of the appropriate age and sex during a similar calendar time. There was a 50% excess in the number of deaths expected from any cause, and twice the number of lung cancer deaths.
1. In Case's mustard gas cohort, what is the contribution to the person years denominator of a man who:
   a) was alive at the end of 1952?
   b) had died during the follow-up period?
2. How would you interpret Case's finding?
3. Can you think of a similar example of a 'one-off exposure' where an epidemiological investigation could provide important information?

Exercise 1.2b
A very different situation existed in the asbestos mine in the Wittenoom Gorge, Western Australia. Here a single employer, Australian Blue Asbestos, had employed a total of 6 220 men over a period of some 20 years[4] for periods ranging from years to a few months. A major series of studies was carried out to determine, among other things, whether there was an association between exposure to asbestos and the occurrence of the pleural cancer, mesothelioma. With regard to the occurrence of mesothelioma over that period, what would you use as the numerator and the denominator?

Exercise 1.3
AIDS (Acquired Immune Deficiency Syndrome) is a well publicised disease and the most important risk factors in Australia include a homosexual lifestyle and/or intravenous drug use. It is one of the infectious diseases which must be notified to the Health Department. In Figure 1.4 the AIDS notification rates are shown for the Sydney health areas.[2] The central Sydney area is roughly around Central Station and includes much high density, low-income housing. Eastern Sydney includes Kings Cross, which is known for its gay community; the other areas correspond to suburban localities.
1. What is the numerator of these notification rates? What is the denominator?
2. Give two reasons why the rates in Kings Cross (eastern Sydney), and around Central Station (central Sydney), might be so much higher than those in the rest of Sydney.

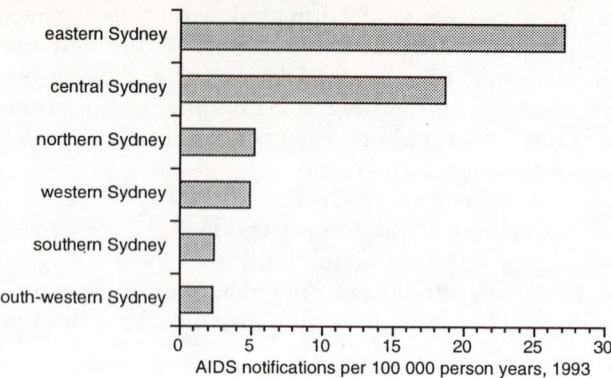

Figure 1.4 *AIDS notification rates per 100 000 person years by Sydney health service areas in 1993.*[2]

ANSWERS

Exercise 1.1

The use of the general population would be misleading because only women, and women who become pregnant, can have a Caesarean section. A population denominator might be 'women aged 15–49', a definition which would at least encompass the number of women in the usually accepted reproductive period.

Exercise 1.2a

1. a) 33 years (from the start of 1930 to the end of 1952).

   b) the amount of time from January 1930 until death.

The interpretation of the finding is that firstly this is an incidence statement in which the numerator is the number of deaths, and the denominator the years over which the men were 'observed'. When the observed number of deaths were compared with that expected from the death rates occurring in the general British population over the same time, a description was available of the risk of premature death in men exposed to mustard gas who had survived some ten years after the war. The situation being described relates to a 'one-off' risk as the exposure only occurred over a fairly short time period. The modern equivalent is the ongoing study of the Hiroshima population exposed to radiation in 1945.

Exercise 1.2b

Similarly to the above example, the numerator was the number of cases of mesothelioma that had occurred in men whilst they were members of the 'at risk population'. This is the time from beginning of employment in the mine to the time of data analysis. The denominator was the accumulated person years spent 'at risk' by these men over the observation period, that is the time spent by each man working in the mine was added up and expressed as a 'person years at risk' denominator. The difference between this and the mustard gas study is that the exposure to asbestos was not a 'one-off' event but rather occurred continuously over an employment period which varied in length from worker to worker. The incidence rate so calculated is a summary of the average rate over the period of operation of the mine and this is why it is sometimes called the 'force of mortality' that was operating.

Exercise 1.3

1. The numerator is the number of individuals fulfilling the criteria for notification as a new case of AIDS. The denominator is the mid-year population of each geographic health area. These are crude rates only because age and gender information is incomplete thus precluding any correction for potential age and gender differences between the areas.
2. People whose lifestyle predisposes them to AIDS tend to gravitate to the central areas of the city and this is particularly likely in the case of certain areas such as Kings Cross. The result of this selective migration from one health area to another is to increase the population 'at risk' of contracting the disease in the central city areas. A second likely reason is also related to selective migration. When a person suspects that he or she may have developed AIDS, a natural tendency might be to move into an area of the city where there would not only be far more chance of finding support groups but also of remaining relatively anonymous. Both these migratory actions would elevate the disease rates in the receiving communities.

CHAPTER TWO
MEASURING HEALTH: MORTALITY

As a physician assesses a patient's health by clinical history and physical examination, so an epidemiologist tries to assess the 'health' of a community. Health itself is difficult to measure, but there are ways of measuring 'illness'. The instruments available are not very precise and include:

1. death rates by age, sex, cause, and calendar year;
2. cancer mortality and morbidity from population-based Cancer Registers (now established in every State);
3. various ad hoc surveys and studies. The Australian Bureau of Statistics (ABS) carries out periodic health surveys, and specific research projects of a data-collecting nature are carried out by researchers, many of which are published in the appropriate scientific literature;
4. hospital separations (deaths, discharges, and transfers) by diagnostic related group (DRG);
5. infectious disease notifications, reported monthly.

There are other data sources of more limited use such as Workers' Compensation statistics. By making comparisons between Australia and other countries, and by looking at trends within Australia, some judgement is possible as to whether Australia is a healthy country. In this chapter we will consider mortality statistics.

CURRENT MORTALITY

For many years the ABS produced a book called *Causes of Death, Australia*. This function has been taken over by the Australian Institute of Health and Welfare which now provides commentary on the statistics produced.[1] The cause of a person's death is taken from the death certificate written by a doctor and this, the underlying cause, is then coded by the ABS in accordance with international rules called the International Classification of Diseases (ICD). These rules are modified periodically and the ninth revision (ICD 9) is currently in use. The strength of the mortality statistics lies in their universality (everyone dies eventually). The fact of death is not in dispute and doctors are legally bound to state the cause of death. The weakness of the system lies in the accuracy with which the cause of death is, or can be, determined. Usually the death certificate is written before an autopsy and is not changed even if a different diagnosis emerges. Even in our largest teaching hospitals, the autopsy rate rarely goes above 20–30% and is zero in nursing homes and similar institutions unless suspicious circumstances are present. Further, it must be admitted that some doctors are rather casual about correctly ascribing the cause of death—especially in the case of older citizens. Nevertheless, the national vital statistics form the foundation by which, paradoxically, the 'health' of a country may be assessed.

Figures 2.1–2.4 show the percentages of the main causes of death by age and sex in Australia in 1992. It is worth remembering the general relative size of the contribution made by these diseases to the all-cause mortality; these causes are shown as percentages of all deaths.

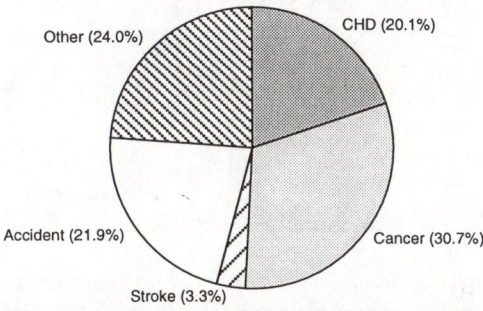

Figure 2.1 *Causes of death in men aged 15–64 in Australia, 1992. Note: CHD (coronary heart disease) refers to the ICD codes 410–414, ischaemic heart disease.*

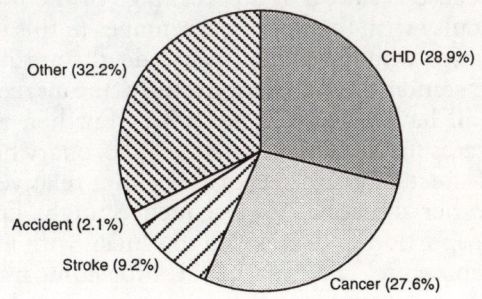

Figure 2.2 *Causes of death in men aged 65 years or more in Australia, 1992.*

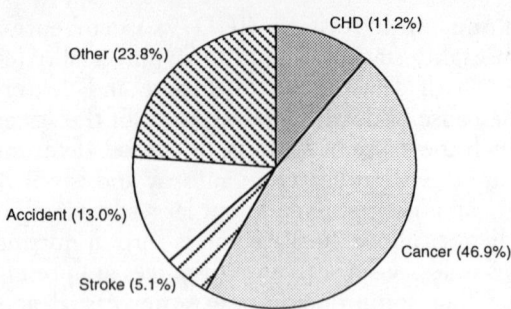

Figure 2.3 *Causes of death in women aged 15–64 in Australia, 1992.*

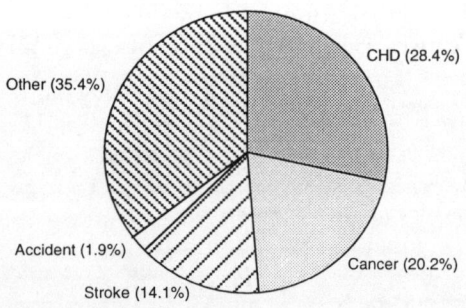

Figure 2.4 *Causes of death in women aged 65 years or more in Australia, 1992.*

An idea of the 'importance' of a particular cause of death in our society is partially conveyed by Figures 2.1–2.4 where the numbers of people dying from that cause is shown as a percentage of the total number of deaths. The difficulty with the use of percentages in this manner is that they cannot indicate whether the all-cause deaths are high or low in relation to some standard. More importantly, the percentages of the different causes all have to add up to 100%. Further, it follows that when the death rates for one disease—such as coronary heart disease—fall, there is of necessity an increase in the relative proportions contributed by other diseases. A consequence might be an apparent increase in the proportion of deaths due to cancer, with much publicity about a 'cancer epidemic'. The use of rates for comparative purposes eliminates this source of error providing that accurate data is available on the size of the denominator, the population at risk.

Cancer Mortality

Figure 2.5 shows some of the most important cancers by site in men and women in Australia, as indicated by mortality statistics. Cancer of the gastrointestinal tract (G–I system) is important in both men and women. Major killers are breast cancer in women and lung cancer in men.

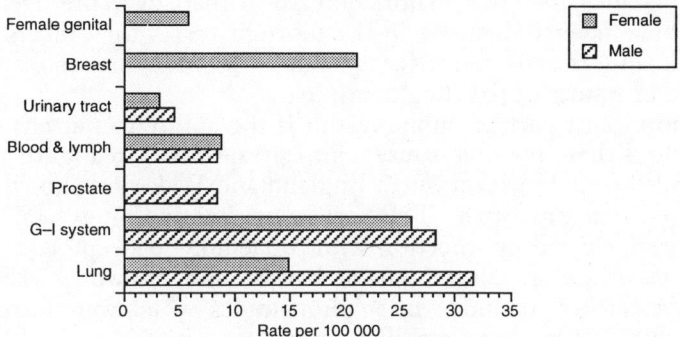

Figure 2.5 *Death rates per 100 000 for selected cancers in men and women aged 35–74, Australia, 1992.*

Changes in Mortality with Time

'Community health', as measured by mortality statistics, is not a static phenomenon but changes in the long, the medium, and in the relatively short-term. For coronary heart disease (CHD), stroke, and accidents, there has been a decline in mortality in both men and women over the last ten years. Figure 2.6 shows the increase that has occurred in suicide of young Australian men since 1981; no such change is apparent in women.[1]

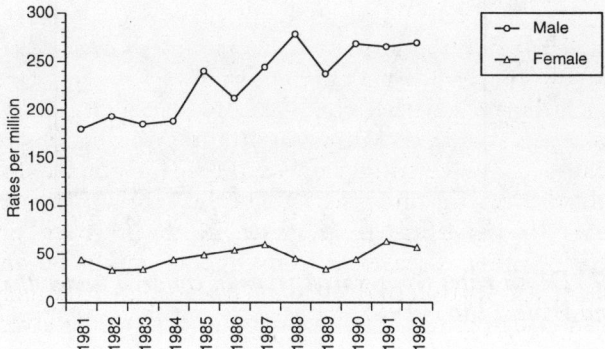

Figure 2.6 *Changes in annual death rates from suicide in men and women aged 15–24, between 1981 and 1992 in Australia.*

13

With regard to all-site cancer, the mortality for both men and women, corrected for age, has shown no particular change over the last ten years. Within this category there have been changes. In men, the most important fall has been in cancer of the stomach and, among a collection of minor increases, the death rate from cancer of the prostate stands out as a major increase in men over the age of 65. There have been reductions in the mortality rates for cancers of the stomach and the reproductive system in women, but a disturbing increase in cancer of the lung continues.

An important part of public health is the ability to put changes in health, and their possible causes, into perspective. In Figure 2.7 the death rates from scarlet fever in England and Wales are shown across a hundred year time span.[2] This very important and often fatal disease of children, caused by infection with β-haemolytic streptococcus, has almost vanished in contemporary Britain and elsewhere. Effective medical treatment includes the sulphonamides, which were introduced in the mid-1930s, and penicillin, introduced in the early 1940s. A glance at the time scale of Figure 2.7 shows that the battle was well and truly over by the time these specific cures were available and it is generally thought that a change in the virulence of the organism was principally responsible. In the case of pulmonary tuberculosis a similar major reduction in mortality occurred over much the same time span and here improvement in nutrition and general health is usually regarded as the reason.

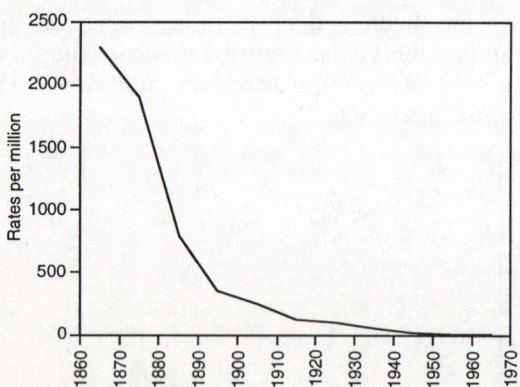

Figure 2.7 *Death rates from scarlet fever in children under the age of 15, England and Wales, 1865–1965.*

Infant Mortality Rates

Countries go through stages of 'healthiness' at different times and at different rates. The main health problems in underdeveloped countries relate to endemic infectious disease and malnutrition; if the country becomes more affluent, concern shifts towards chronic degenerative disease and psychiatric morbidity. If a single index were to be nominated as a 'marker' of this progress it would be the infant mortality rate.

$$\text{Infant Mortality Rate (IMR)} = \frac{\text{deaths in babies under one year}}{\text{live births in that year}} \times 1\,000$$

The IMR in Australia, which was 104 in 1901, was 7 in 1992. By way of contrast, the Aboriginal IMR in 1992 was 25 in South Australia, and 27 in the Northern Territory.[3]

'What was the cause of death?'

When we look at the patterns of mortality between countries, or between Australian States, we are dependent upon the quality of the data written on the death certificates and on the system of coding used by the Australian Bureau of Statistics to label the 'cause of death'. Figure 2.8 is an example of the style of death certificate that follows World Health Organisation recommendations, and this is used in Australia as in most countries. The mortality statistics published describe for each death the 'underlying cause', which is defined as the disease or injury which initiated the train of morbid events leading directly to death. Such underlying causes would be derived from the death certificate as in the following asterisked examples:

Case A:　a. hepatic failure
Part I　　　b. bile duct obstruction
　　　　　　c. carcinoma of the pancreas*

Case B:　a. cerebral haemorrhage
Part I　　　b. hypertension
　　　　　　c. chronic pyelonephritis*

Case A refers to a person whose final demise was due to the fact that his liver had ceased to function. However, the liver did not fail of itself—it failed because the bile duct, the function of which is to allow waste products to drain away into the bowel, became blocked. To follow this train of events a little further, the bile duct did not become blocked because of some problem of the duct itself (such as an impacted gallstone), but rather because of a cancer of the pancreas. Due to the anatomical proximity of the pancreas to the duct, a pancreatic growth can compress the duct and prevent the liver from

15

doing its job. The underlying cause is thus the cancer (carcinoma). Similarly, in Case B the sequence is long-standing disease of the kidneys causing high blood pressure which, in turn, is directly responsible for the immediate cause of death, namely a cerebral haemorrhage or stroke.

<table>
<tr><td colspan="2" align="center">**Cause of Death**</td><td>Approximate
interval between
onset and death</td></tr>
<tr><td>**PART 1**
Disease or
condition directly</td><td>(a) ....</td><td>...................</td></tr>
<tr><td>leading to death.</td><td align="center">due to or as a consequence of</td><td></td></tr>
<tr><td>Antecedent
causes (morbid
conditions, if any</td><td>(b) ....</td><td>...................</td></tr>
<tr><td>giving rise to the
above mentioned</td><td align="center">due to or as a consequence of</td><td></td></tr>
<tr><td>cause, stating the
underlying
condition first.</td><td>(c) ....</td><td>...................</td></tr>
<tr><td>**PART 2**
Other significant
conditions
contributing to
the death but not</td><td>...</td><td>...................</td></tr>
<tr><td>related to the
disease or causing it.</td><td>...</td><td>...................</td></tr>
</table>

Figure 2.8 *Style of death certificate in use in NSW.*

One of the hospital jobs of a first year resident is to complete such death certificates and sometimes the certificate is written out less logically.

Case C:

Part I	a. nephrectomy
Part II	b. carcinoma of the kidney*

Here the coder would take what was written in Part II as the underlying cause because the reason that the kidney was removed (nephrectomy) was the presence of cancer.

EXERCISES

Exercise 2.1

1. How do you think that a death certificate (underlying cause of death) should be completed for each of the cases described below?

Case A: Mrs AB 59 years

Admitted to hospital with one hour central chest pain radiating down the left arm. She had a past history of chest pain on exertion and had been trying to lose weight for many years.

On admission she was obese, pulse rate 100, BP 140/90. There was a third heart sound. Her chest was clear. ECG showed ischaemic ST-T changes in the anterior chest leads and Q waves developed on these leads on the next day. Cardiac enzymes were elevated.

She developed slight shortness of breath and was slow to mobilise. Seven days after admission she developed sudden shortness of breath, coughed up blood-stained sputum and died shortly afterwards.

Post mortem showed a healing recent anterior myocardial infarct and a large pulmonary embolus occluding most of the vascular bed of the right lung with an associated infarction of the right lower lobe.

Case B: Mr JL 67 years

Admitted to hospital with increasing nausea, cough and breathlessness, he had been treated for congestive cardiac failure five years previously and on admission was taking Lanoxin, Aldomet, Serepax and Nuelin. Examination showed dyspnoea at rest, pulse rate 110, BP 140/80, JVP raised 8 cm. His heart was enlarged and he was in atrial fibrillation. He had gross ankle oedema and bilateral basal crepitations. His liver was 5 cm enlarged and not tender.

He was treated with diuretics, vasodilators and anticoagulants. Sputum culture grew Klebsiella pneumoniae and he was started on antibiotics. ECG showed small voltage complexes and atrial fibrillation. There was also evidence of an old anterior infarction. Chest X-ray showed an enlarged heart and consolidation in the right lower lobe.

His sputum production and ankle oedema declined somewhat but he remained dyspnoeic; the chest signs remained the same and his chest X-ray did not improve. Despite continuing treatment he died.

You may like to compare your ideas with those of doctors in practice. Seventy-five doctors in each of the Australian States and New Zealand, and a further 27 in the Northern Territory, were asked to complete a death certificate on these cases (and eight others).[4] About 70% of doctors responded; Tables 2.1 and 2.2 show that considerable variation was observed in what was written on the death certificates. This is quite surprising because medical training is fairly uniform throughout Australasia. The State coding offices were then asked to code a diagnosis for each certificate in their usual manner and, perhaps surprisingly, variation in the attributed cause of death was still present.

Table 2.1 Percentage of certificates coded to main causes of death (**Case A**).

	Acute myocardial infarction (%)	*Pulmonary embolus* (%)	*Other diagnoses* (%)
New South Wales	78	18	4
Victoria	76	10	14
Queensland	75	13	13
South Australia	78	10	12
Western Australia	90	0	10
Tasmania	100	0	0
Northern Territory	84	5	11
New Zealand	97	0	3

Table 2.2 Percentage of certificates coded to main cause of death (**Case B**).

	Ischaemic heart disease (%)	*Other heart disease* (%)	*Pneumonia* (%)	*Other diagnoses* (%)
New South Wales	52	16	28	4
Victoria	41	20	29	10
Queensland	46	19	27	8
South Australia	44	24	22	10
Western Australia	53	14	20	12
Tasmania	53	41	0	7
Northern Territory	42	21	32	5
New Zealand	43	12	38	8

2. What do you think might be the implications of these results for:
   a) a doctor in practice?
   b) studies of inter-State variations in mortality patterns?
   c) studies of international differences in mortality patterns?
   Do you think that anything should be done about the situation?
   If so, what?

ANSWERS

Exercise 2.1

1. Compare your answers to those of the doctors, given in Tables 2.1 and 2.2.
2. a) Probably none at all!
   b) Differences in mortality between Australian States of a significant degree and in important conditions could set people wondering about differences in the environments and cultures of the States in question. Hypotheses would be generated and much money and time wasted. If diagnostic fashions varied not only between States, but from time to time within States, then our knowledge of trends in disease processes, the success or otherwise of broad health strategies, and the relationship between service provision and health would be based on misleading data.
   c) Generally as above but here we would be comparing our country with others and could be drawing the same false conclusions.

CHAPTER THREE
MEASURING HEALTH: MORBIDITY

B ecause mortality data are readily available in published form, they tend to colour our view of which diseases are 'important', and we can easily underrate those conditions which cause much unhappiness but are not lethal.

In 1993 a study was reported by Britt and colleagues[1] of consultations in New South Wales and Queensland general practices in both metropolitan and country areas. Figure 3.1 shows the percentages of the six most frequent reasons given by patients for their consultation with a metropolitan general practitioner. The pattern of 'health problems' perceived by people shows no resemblance to the common causes of mortality in Australia shown in the previous chapter.

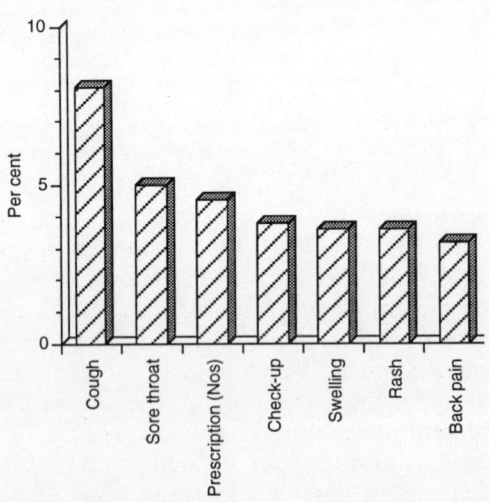

Figure 3.1 *Reasons given by patients for consulting metropolitan general practitioners.*[1]

In contrast, Figure 3.2 shows the six leading 'problems' as categorised by the general practitioner following the consultation. Whilst this classification is in terms of what is believed to be the underlying pathology, the distribution suggests a priority list which would be different again from that made on the basis of death rates. It is easy to see why those who are responsible for allocating health resources, or even those who design health studies curricula, have difficulty in deciding what is important and where the money should go!

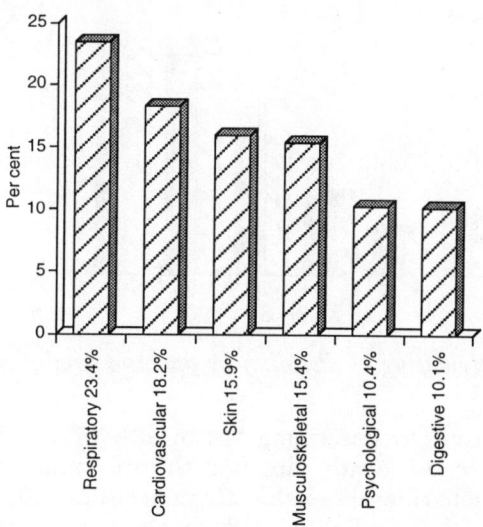

Figure 3.2 *Reasons for general practice consultation—all ages and both sexes.*[1]

Morbidity can be described not only in terms of pathology but also as the effects of the functioning of that pathology on people, which is perhaps of more importance in the social context. Disability may be defined as the disturbance of 'customarily expected activity, behaviour or performance' due to the presence of a disease process. Measurements of the amount of disability in the community are made by planned surveys of the population such as those carried out by the Australian Bureau of Statistics in 1981, 1988 and 1993. In these surveys, disability was defined rather differently as the presence of one or more specified medical conditions which had been present (or expected to be present) for at least six months. On this definition it was estimated that 18% of Australians were disabled in some way. The proportion of those disabled varies with age and gender (see Figure 3.3), by degree of disability, and by its cause. In the light of the data shown in Figures 3.1

and 3.2 it will come as no surprise that the most frequently reported source of disability lay in the musculoskeletal system (4.9%) with the next being hearing loss (2.6%) and mental disorders (2%).[2] It is information of this type that enables State health departments to plan for equitable distribution of resources and to justify new developments in health care to finance divisions, often with quite different agendas.

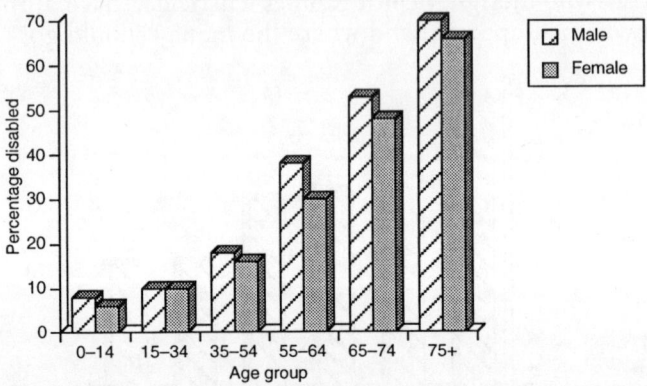

Figure 3.3 *Prevalence of disability by age and gender in an Australian population, 1993.*[2]

Another approach to describing the health of a community is to estimate neither the death rate nor the morbidity, but rather the prevalence of behavioural or other characteristics which are known to be precursors of disease. Table 3.1 shows the prevalence of certain risk factors, or disease precursors, in men living in the Hunter Valley.[3] By Australian standards these data do not indicate a healthy community.

Table 3.1 Prevalence of selected 'risk factors' in Hunter Valley men, 1989.[3]

Age group	20–29	30–39	40–49	50–59	60–69
Hypertension	2.8%	9.2%	20.8%	32.2%	39.6%
Current smoker	25.7%	32.1%	28.0%	25.7%	18.3%
Drinks alcohol 5+ days a week	42.8 %	23.7%	26.6%	28.0%	33.0%
Number of subjects	35	131	207	214	321

Setting Priorities

One of the important functions of epidemiology is to provide the information needed for governments to set priorities in health care and research. In a reality of finite budgets and human resources it is helpful to have some idea of what health goals are desirable, which are attainable, and how progress in achieving them could be monitored. The World Health Organization began the task by setting the worldwide goal of 'Health for all by the year 2000!' Using epidemiological data, the Australian Department of Health made an initial response in 1985,[4] a response which was supplemented by a more sophisticated approach in 1993 by Nutbeam and colleagues.[5] As an example of the way priorities can be set and progress towards goals measured, we can select from Nutbeam's list one condition for study, namely HIV/AIDS.

The first element is that the disease must be a serious health problem and in Australia it is estimated that some 15 000 people are HIV positive, of whom more than 3 400 had developed AIDS by June 1992. Secondly, there needs to be some well founded belief that the condition is amenable to prevention. In Australia the preventive strategies that have been devised and implemented have been associated with a low (by international standards) infection rate via intravenous drug use, and a slowing of the epidemic progress among homosexual and bisexual men. Finally, for effective and efficient intervention it is necessary that subpopulations at greater risk of contracting the disease in question can be defined.

Goal: To reduce the incidence and impact of HIV/AIDS.
Target: Priority population—sexually active people and IV drug users.
Aim: To reduce the incidence of HIV by 40% by the year 2 000.
Baseline: It is currently estimated that there are 600 new HIV infections per annum or an annual rate of about 3.5/100 000.

EXERCISES

Exercise 3.1
One of the health goals for Australia is to reduce the incidence of suicide attempts. In the context of this goal can you list four subpopulations in Australia that seem to be at particular risk of suicide?
1. Answer from your general knowledge.
2. Give data-supported reasons for your selection of subpopulations.

Exercise 3.2
Table 3.2 is taken from the annual mortality statistics of the ABS.[6,7] It shows the number of deaths from stomach cancer in Australia in men at certain ages in 1981 and 1992. For the purpose of this exercise only, assume that the population size and age structure did not change significantly between these periods.

Table 3.2 Deaths from stomach cancer (ICD 151) in Australian men aged 45 years or more.

Age group	1981	1992
45–64	239	187
65+	617	546

1. Which age group has contributed most to the observed reduction in mortality:
   a) in absolute terms?
   b) proportionally?
2. Under what circumstances would (a) or (b) be the appropriate measure of change?

Exercise 3.3

The case-fatality rate is an oft quoted disease charactistic, being the number of deaths from the disease divided by the number of people who acquire the disease during the same time period.

Each year the NSW Health Department reports the number of people who are admitted to a hospital with a diagnosis of intentional self harm.[8] The ABS also records the number of people in the State who have died with the cause of death being labelled 'suicide' in each year.[9] If we divide the number of suicides by the number of attempted suicides (both successful and unsuccessful), as indicated by hospital admission, is the result a valid index of the case-fatality rate of attempted suicide?

ANSWERS

Exercise 3.1

1. General knowledge should be adequate to reach at least some of the same conclusions as Nutbeam and his colleagues on the question of subpopulations at most risk:
   - young adults 20–25 years of age;
   - all Aboriginals and Torres Straits Islanders;
   - young people 15–19 years living in rural communities;
   - older, widowed males.
2. To support (or challenge) in a quantitative manner these subpopulation selections it will be necessary to search the literature by way of Medline or other appropriate database.

Exercise 3.2

The differences between 1981 and 1992 for the 45–64 age group is 52 people (absolute) representing a 21.8% reduction in mortality. For the 65+ age group the absolute reduction was 71 deaths representing an 11.5% mortality reduction.

Both ways of expressing change have their appropriate place but only the absolute figures can tell us about the importance of the change in the health of the community. The 21.8% change noted in the 45–64 year old group suggests that something, perhaps diet, has changed in the community and investigation of stomach cancer from an epidemiological perspective might well be a productive research project. On the other hand, 12 688 men aged 45–64 died in 1992 and a reduction in the number of stomach cancer deaths by 52 therefore does not indicate much of a change in the overall health of the community.

Exercise 3.3

Suicides in a population such as that of New South Wales, over a designated time period, may be illustrated as in the Venn diagram (Figure 3.4). The large circle includes all suicide attempts in the community, only some of which were serious enough for the person to be admitted to hospital, and these appear as one of the inner circles. The small circle represents deaths from suicide, most of which never reach hospital with the person being dead when found. Whilst we do have a numerator for a case-fatality ratio—the number of deaths—no estimate is possible of the denominator which is the total number of suicide attempts in the community. For this reason the ratio suggested is not an appropriate indicator.

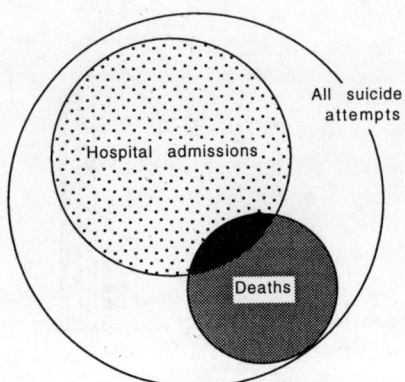

Figure 3.4 *Schematic representation of the distribution of suicides, both successful and unsuccessful, in the community.*

CHAPTER FOUR

MORTALITY & MORBIDITY: COMPARISONS OF TIME & PLACE

Comparisons of disease rates between different cities, different countries, and different times, are very important in epidemiology. As far as possible we want to compare 'like with like' and the variable usually most in need of control is that of age. A crude annual death rate is calculated by dividing the number of deaths that occur in a year, by the population 'at risk'; in 1981 the all cause crude death rate for women in Australia was 646 per 100 000. In 1992 this crude rate had increased to 656 per 100 000 and it would appear that the state of women's health, as measured by mortality statistics,[1] had deteriorated. Another way of looking at the mortality statistics, however, is to consider the death rate within age groups, where the numerator is the number of deaths in women of a certain age and the denominator the population of that age. These are known as 'age-specific rates' and are shown graphically in Figure 4.1 for women in 1981 and in 1992.

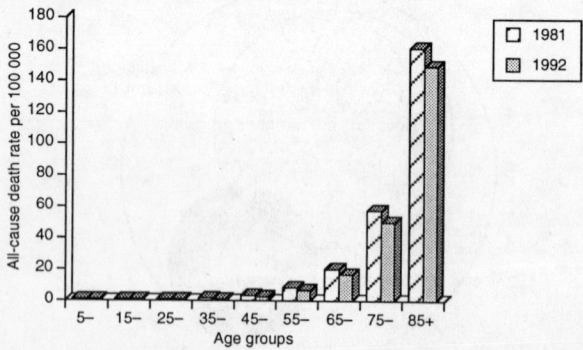

Figure 4.1 *Age-specific all-cause death rates for Australian women in 1981 and in 1992.*[1]

As is illustrated by the figure, although the crude death rate has increased, consideration of age-specific rates shows a consistent improvement across the board within each age group in the 1992 rates. This seems a puzzle; if we think of the crude rate as some kind of average of the age-specific rates, it seems hard to see how the crude rate goes up while all the age-specific rates go down. The reason is that the death rate rises very sharply with age and hence the crude rate is very sensitive to the proportion of older people in the population. Over the period 1981–1992 the age distribution of Australian women has shifted to the right due to declining death rates and to falling birth rates. So the 1992 crude rate is more heavily influenced by the rates in older women (see Exercise 4.2). For the same reason we would expect the crude death rate from a retirement area like Queensland's Gold Coast to be higher than that from a newly developed suburb in Melbourne or Sydney. To make a comparison between such areas, it would be necessary to compare age-specific rates or, more conveniently, to 'standardise' the rates for age. Such standardisation is also appropriate for morbidity rates.

In a national survey, workers in the Australian petroleum industry[2] were asked whether they had ever had a skin cancer. The proportion of positive replies, by age, is shown in Figure 4.2 and is strongly age related.

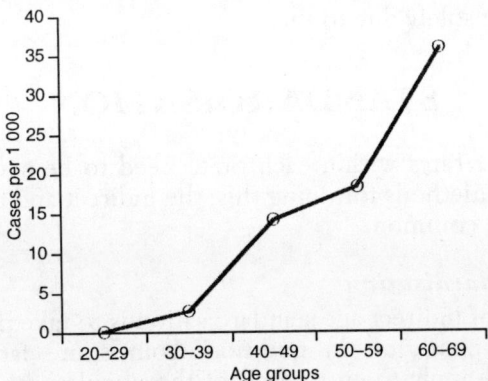

Figure 4.2 *Lifetime prevalence of self-reported non-melanotic skin cancer in petroleum workers by age group.*

Another analysis carried out (see Figure 4.3) showed considerable variation between Australian States in the occurrence of skin cancer in petroleum industry workers living in those States.

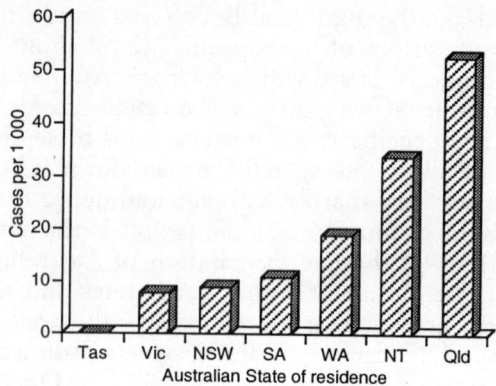

Figure 4.3 *Lifetime prevalence of self-reported non-melanotic skin cancer, by State of residence.*

We now have two pieces of information. Firstly, skin cancer is strongly age-related which is inevitable in a measure of 'lifetime prevalence'. Secondly, it appears to be related to State of residence. To conclude that a true State effect exists, it is necessary to confirm that the apparent difference is not due entirely to differing age structures in the different States. If the workers in Queensland happened to be much older than those in Victoria, the difference between the rates in the two States could be solely due to this.

STANDARDISATION

The prevalence rates within each State need to be age standardised. There are two methods for doing this, the indirect and the direct. The former is more common.

Indirect standardisation

The principle of indirect age standardisation is to take the age-specific rates for the condition in question from some larger reference population and apply them to each of the populations that are to be compared. The result will be the number of cases or events which would have been 'expected' in each age group had those reference rates applied. The sum of the expected number may then be compared with the number of cases that were actually 'observed'. For a population to be used as the reference, its appropriate event rates need to be known, and for mortality comparisons the Australian death rates are usual in Australian studies. In the petroleum industry example, since there is no appropriate population whose non-melanotic skin cancer rates are known, the reference rates will have to be those applying to the total, all-State population of petroleum workers. The procedure is as follows:

1. take the age-specific rates for the whole population of workers (Table 4.1);
2. apply these rates to the population of each State separately, thus producing an 'expected' number of cases as if the rates for the whole population applied equally in each State;
3. for each State, calculate the ratio of the total number of 'observed' cases to the total number of 'expected' cases.

The result is known as a standardised morbidity ratio (SMR). If the age-specific rates for each State were identical to that of the whole population of workers, then the SMR for each State would be 1, that is, the number of cases 'expected' in each State would be identical to the number 'observed'. Note that the abbreviation SMR may refer to standardised mortality ratio or standardised morbidity ratio, but generally the context resolves any ambiguity.

Table 4.1 Data for calculation of standardised morbidity ratio of Victorian petroleum industry workers (unpublished data).

1 *Age* *group*	*2* *Whole* *population* *rates per 10^3*	*3* *Age* *distribution* *(Vic)*	*4* *'Expected'* *no. of cases* *(Vic)*	*5* *Observed* *no. of cases* *(Vic)*
15–24	0.00	77	0.00	
25–34	2.59	777	2.01	
35–44	13.94	922	12.85	
45–54	18.15	700	12.71	
55–64	35.71	313	11.18	
15–64		*2 789*	*38.75*	*17*

Key

Column 1 = age groups
Column 2 = skin cancer rates for all workers in all States combined
Column 3 = age distribution of Victorian workers
Column 4 = number of cases 'expected' in Victoria when the age-specific rates in column 2 are applied to the appropriate age group of Victorian workers (column 3); (ie column 2 × column 3)
Column 5 = number of cases actually reported from Victoria

The SMR is calculated as observed/expected = (17/38.75) = 0.44.

If we calculate the SMR for each State in the same way, we still see a considerable difference between the States (Table 4.2). The addition of a new piece of information, namely the average hours of daily sunshine in each State capital, completes Table 4.2. There is a correlation between prevalence of skin cancer and average hours of sunshine and, because we have standardised for age, we can be certain that the observed variation in SMR by State is not solely explicable in terms of age differences.

Table 4.2 Standardised morbidity ratios (SMR) for non-melanotic skin cancer prevalence by State, and average daily sunshine hours in State capitals.

State	Vic	NSW	SA	WA	NT	Qld
SMR	0.44	0.55	0.68	1.29	2.44	3.47
Sunshine hrs per day	5.70	6.70	7.90	7.90	8.50	7.50

This is the process of indirect standardisation where a standard, or reference, age-specific disease rate from a large and more stable population is being applied to a subset of that population.

A more typical example of the use of the method comes from a recent study of mortality in New South Wales coalminers[3] in which death was the event of interest. The population at risk consisted of all miners who had joined the industry between the beginning of 1973 and the end of 1992. State death registers were examined to determine the number of miners who had died and these became the numerator of the death rates, the denominator being calculated as person years at risk (PYR). During the follow-up period, 491 miners died and the death rates for all cause deaths, and for deaths from specific causes, were standardised for age by the indirect method. The age-specific rates for New South Wales were used as the reference. Some results are shown in Table 4.3. Note that SMR in this context means standardised mortality ratio, because the event of interest is death.

Table 4.3 SMR for deaths by all cause and selected causes in NSW coalminers 1973–92.

Cause	Observed	Expected	SMR
All causes	491	642.85	0.76
Cancer	92	118.71	0.78
Heart disease	90	135.21	0.67
Cerebrovascular disease	15	23.15	0.65
Respiratory disease	13	17.83	0.73
Motor vehicle accidents	94	80.63	1.17
Other accidents	84	52.38	1.60
Suicide	47	61.86	0.76
Other external causes	10	11.34	0.88

For 'all causes', and for a number of specific causes, the numbers of deaths that were observed have been compared with the numbers expected had the rates experienced by the general New South Wales population applied. Because these deaths were accumulated across a 20-year time span, account had to be taken of changing rates in the reference population so the 'expected deaths' were calculated in five-year blocks of calendar time against the appropriate State rates of that time. The table shows that, among other things, the all cause death rate for miners was only 76% of that experienced by the general population whereas the deaths from non-motor vehicle ('other') accidents was elevated to 60% above that of the reference population. Because of the age standardisation these differences are not due to different age structures in the study and reference populations.

If we wished to compare death rates in Newcastle with those in Perth, we could apply the age-specific death rates from the whole Australian population to the appropriate age strata in each city. The result would be the number of deaths in Newcastle and in Perth 'expected' were the Australian rates to apply, and we would be able to compare these numbers with the number of deaths that actually occurred. For each city separately, the ratio would be the standardised mortality ratio, and thus an age standardised comparison of death rates would be possible.

Direct standardisation

Generally indirect standardisation is used, but occasionally another method is used. Instead of taking the death rates from the reference population and applying these to the various populations of interest, in the method known as direct standardisation, the rates observed in the sub-populations are applied to the reference population. For each sub-population one then has the number of deaths which would have been 'expected' in the reference population had the sub-population's rates applied. Division by the number of people in the reference population gives a standardised mortality rate.

Expected deaths ÷ Reference population = a standardised rate

Multiplication by a convenient number (for example 10^6) may be carried out, to give whole numbers (standardised rates per million). This method was adopted by the Australian Institute of Health and Welfare in reporting death rates from various causes across time as in Figure 4.4 where death rates for motor vehicle accidents in Australia from 1981 to 1992 have been directly standardised against the national population.[1] The fall is marked and coincides with major efforts to improve road safety. Whether the latter are responsible for the fall in road accident deaths cannot be determined solely from the statistics presented.

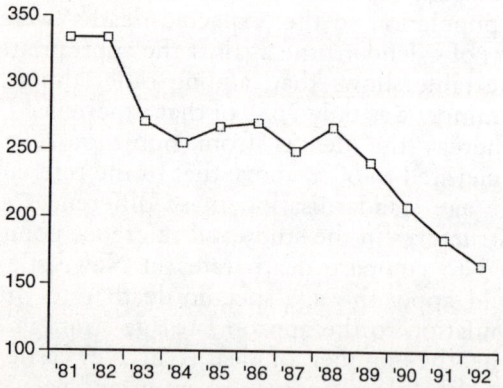

Figure 4.4 *Age standardised mortality rates for motor vehicle accidents in Australia 1981–92.[1]*

EXERCISES

Exercise 4.1

In 1981 a study of coronary heart disease (CHD) in the British army was reported[4] and in Table 4.4 the relevant numbers of deaths in both officers and 'other ranks' are shown. These were observed over a period of five years. In addition, the general male population CHD annual death rates are shown.

Table 4.4 CHD death rates in the general male population of England and Wales, in British army officers and in 'other ranks'.

Age group	CHD general pop.: rates per 100 000 per year	Officers CHD observed (five years)	Officers Pop. in 1 000s	Officers Rate per 100 000 per year	Other Ranks CHD observed (five years)	Other Ranks Pop. in 1 000s	Other Ranks Rate per 100 000 per year
15–19	0.2	0	0.1		0	25.3	
20–24	0.7	0	1.8		4	45.2	
25–29	2.9	0	2.6		10	32.9	
30–34	10.2	0	2.3		26	17.6	
35–39	33.5	2	2.7		36	12.1	
40–44	94.2	6	3.0		19	4.3	
45–49	204.3	14	2.7		11	1.1	
50–54	371.9	19	1.5		2	0.3	

1. What are the crude death rates (that is all age) for the officers and for the 'other ranks' respectively? What does this suggest? Note that the observation period was five years, so that to obtain the 'per year' rates the population must be multiplied by five.
2. Calculate the age-specific death rates in officers and in 'other ranks'.
3. Compare the age-specific rates. What light does this shed on the difference in crude rates?
4. Using the data that have been given, calculate the standardised mortality ratios for the officers and 'other ranks'. Annual rates are given, so that to obtain the 'expected' numbers over the five-year period, it is necessary to multiply by five.

Exercise 4.2

Table 4.5 shows the age distributions and numbers of deaths in women in Australia in 1981 and in 1992. Use direct standardisation with 1992 as the reference population to compare the mortality experience in the two years. How does this help to resolve the paradox referred to in the text?

Table 4.5 Deaths (all cause) and populations by age, women in Australia in 1981 and in 1992.

Age group	1981 Deaths	1981 Population	1992 Deaths	1992 Population
0–4	1 203	556 400	948	623 262
5–14	241	1 265 789	178	1 230 546
15–24	589	1 278 293	518	1 351 222
25–44	1 655	2 103 778	1 921	2 730 509
45–64	7 789	1 429 146	6 947	1 693 378
65–84	24 828	76 989	29 730	1 026 548
85 +	11 995	74 805	17 301	116 169
all ages	48 300	7 476 200	57 543	8 771 634

ANSWERS

Exercise 4.1

1. Crude rate for officers   = 49.1/10^5/year.
   Crude rate for other ranks = 15.6/10^5/year.
This certainly suggests that officers have a greater risk of a heart attack than the rank and file soldiers. Immediate thoughts might take the line of 'the stress of command' and so forth.
2. See the following table.

Table 4.6 Age-specific death rates from CHD per 10^5, British Army.[4]

Age	15–19	20–24	25–29	30–34	35–39	40–44	45–49	50–54
Officers	0	0	0	0	14.8	40.0	103.7	253.3
Other ranks	0	1.8	6.1	29.5	59.5	88.4	200.0	133.3

3. From the crude rates it would appear that the officers have a much higher death rate than the soldiers. When the age-specific rates are examined the opposite appears to be true, with the exception of the 50–54 year group where the very small number of deaths in 'other ranks' (two) makes this a most unreliable rate. The paradox is due to the grossly unequal age distribution of the two populations with the other ranks having a much higher proportion of young men. Thus, in the crude rate for 'other ranks', the denominator is loaded with

young men with low mortality and for this reason appears lower in comparison to the officers.

4. Calculation of SMR.

Table 4.7 Calculation of the SMR for CHD in officers and 'other ranks' in the British army.

Age group	Officers			Other ranks		
	Population (000s)	Ref. rate (per 10⁵)	Expected (5 yrs)	Population (000s)	Ref. rate (per 10⁵)	Expected (5 yrs)
15–19	0.1	0.2	0	25.3	0.2	0.25
20–24	1.8	0.7	0.06	45.2	0.7	1.58
25–29	2.6	2.9	0.38	32.9	2.9	4.77
30–34	2.3	10.2	1.17	17.6	10.2	8.98
35–39	2.7	33.5	4.52	12.1	33.5	20.27
40–44	3.0	94.2	14.13	4.3	94.2	20.25
45–49	2.7	204.3	27.58	1.1	204.3	11.24
50–54	1.5	371.9	27.89	0.3	371.9	5.58
Total			75.73			72.92

SMR officers = 41/75.73 = 0.54
SMR other ranks = 108/72.94 = 1.48

The reasons for the excess mortality in the soldiers are not clear. Perhaps the difference can be attributed to social class which presumably acts as a marker for behaviour associated with heart disease risk factors such as cigarette smoking.

Exercise 4.2

In Table 4.8 the age-specific rates of the two populations are shown. The 'deaths expected' column shows the number of deaths 'expected' if the age-specific rates for 1981 are applied to 1992 as the reference population.

Table 4.8 Calculation of a standardised death rate.

Age	1981 Deaths	1981 Pop.	1981 Rate per 10 000	1992 Deaths	1992 Pop.	1992 Rate per 10 000	Deaths expected
0–4	1 203	556 400	21.6	948	623 262	15.2	1 346.2
5–14	241	1 265 789	1.9	178	1 230 546	1.4	233.8
15–24	589	1 278 293	4.9	518	1 351 222	3.8	662.1
25–44	1 655	2 103 778	7.9	1 921	2 730 509	7.0	2 157.1
45–64	7 789	1 429 146	54.5	6 947	1 693 378	41.0	9 228.9
65–84	24 828	767 989	323.3	29 730	1 026 548	289.6	33 188.3
85 +	11 995	74 805	1 603.5	17 301	116 169	1 489.3	18 627.7
Total	*48 360*	*7 476 200*		*57 543*	*8 771 634*		*65 444.1*

The standardised death rate for 1981 (direct method) using 1992 as the reference population = 65 444.1 / 8 771 634 = 74.6 per 10 000. This rate may be compared to the 1992 crude rate which was 57 543 / 8 771 634 = 65.6 per 10 000. (Note that the 'standardised' death rate for 1992, using 1992 as the reference, is simply the 1992 crude rate.) Now it becomes clear that, after appropriate adjustment for age, the 1981 mortality experience was worse than that in 1992; the opposite impression conveyed by the difference in crude rates is merely a reflection of the differing age structures of the 1981 and 1992 Australian female populations.

CHAPTER FIVE

RISK & CAUSE

An important function of epidemiology lies in the identification of factors that indicate that certain individuals are at greater risk than others of developing a particular disease. It is necessary to consider how such risk may be measured, because measurement is of fundamental importance when decisions are being made about whether a particular risk is 'acceptable' or not. This notion of measuring risk applies to a wide range of personal characteristics and behaviours, such as blood pressure or cigarette smoking, and also to environmental factors, such as exposure to chemicals in the workplace. Some 'risk factors' are preventable; others, such as age, are not and should be regarded more as indicators.

The community has to somehow strike a balance between a risk (such as that due to smoking) on the one hand and freedom of choice on the other. A risk (such as exposure to asbestos) has to be balanced against the gain from having a most useful building material. Views on what is acceptable change. In the 1960s, the risk taking associated with the Maralinga bomb tests was (presumably) regarded as a military necessity. In many countries today the risk taking associated with nuclear power is regarded as an economic necessity.

Risk is measured in a number of ways in epidemiology but the two fundamental measures are known as relative risk and attributable risk.

RELATIVE RISK

The relative risk may be defined as:

> the ratio of the rate at which disease occurs in people who
> are exposed to the presumed cause, to the rate among those
> not so exposed.

An example of the use of relative risk is given in a study by Doll and colleagues in a South Wales nickel refinery.[1] Here the purpose was to explore the risk of death from lung cancer as a consequence of exposure to nickel. The death rates of those men who had worked in the refinery before 1925 are compared in Table 5.1 with the age-specific death rates experienced by the male population of England and Wales during the appropriate calendar time periods. Here, as is frequently done in occupational studies, the general population is regarded as not exposed to the presumed causal factor.

Table 5.1 Age adjusted lung cancer death rates per 1 000 person years at risk in exposed and non-exposed populations.[1]

Exposure status	*Death rates per 1 000 PYR**
Nickel workers (employed before 1925)	17.9
Non-exposed general male population	2.4

* PYR = person years at risk

Relative Risk = 17.9/2.4 = 7.5. This means that the risk of death from lung cancer to nickel workers employed before 1925 was 7.5 times that of the general population.

Another example of the use of relative risk comes from the mortality study of Australian Vietnam war veterans[2] (Table 5.2). Here also, because the veterans were followed up for various time periods, the denominator of the death rates was expressed as person years at risk.

Table 5.2 All cause death rates in Australian Vietnam war veterans compared with the rates in those servicemen who did not serve in Vietnam.

	Deaths	*PYR*	*Death rates per 1 000 PYR*
Veterans	260	225 317	1.15
Non-veterans	263	294 083	0.89

Relative Risk = 1.15/0.89 = 1.29

In the above examples the data came from ongoing observations on defined populations at risk. In the context of case–control studies, for reasons which will be discussed in a later chapter, another way of expressing risk will be required.

In each of the examples a single presumed causal factor, being exposed to nickel or being a veteran, was analysed. In reality, of course, a disease is often the result of the operation of several different causes which may interact. Consider the relative risks for lung cancer in three groups of men in whom two causal factors are operating, smoking and exposure to asbestos.[3] The group with whom the other three are compared is the baseline group, non-smokers not exposed to asbestos.

Non-smoker, not exposed to asbestos   RR = 1.0 (baseline)
Non-smoker, exposed to asbestos   RR = 5.2
Smoker, not exposed to asbestos   RR = 10.9
Smoker, exposed to asbestos   RR = 53.2

The interaction of these two factors is not one of the simple addition of one risk to another but is multiplicative, as is shown in Figure 5.1. Such multiplication of risks is usual, rather than otherwise, and has obvious implications not only for preventive health counselling, but also in legal wrangles over compensation claims. 'What was the real cause of the lung cancer, asbestos exposure at work or cigarette smoking in his own time?'

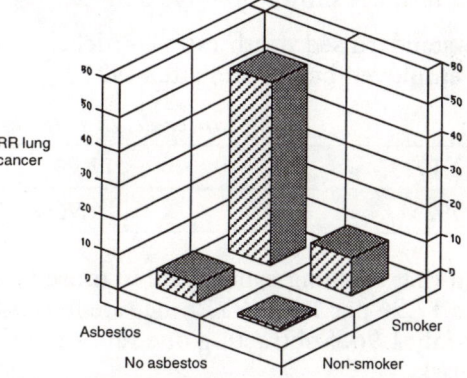

Figure 5.1 *Relative risks for lung cancer in groups of men classified by smoking habit and by exposure to asbestos.*

Being a ratio, the relative risk cannot give any idea of the size of the problem in absolute terms. The relative risk of developing angiosarcoma of the liver in men exposed to vinyl chloride monomer is 250 but, because the disease is so rare, only a few hundred or so cases have ever been reported. To get some feel for absolute numbers we need another term, attributable risk.

ATTRIBUTABLE RISK

Attributable risk may be defined as:

the difference between the rates at which disease occurs in people who are exposed, and in people who are not so exposed.

The public health importance of attributable risk is that it gives us a measure of the incidence of disease in exposed individuals which may be attributed to that exposure. Conversely, it indicates the reduction in disease which may be expected from removal of the exposure. Such information enables the proposers of, say, a health promotion campaign, to make a much stronger case for government or other funding if it can be sold in terms of number of lives that could be 'saved' and the consequent dollar savings to the community. In a clinical context, it is often helpful to be able to explain the meaning of a health risk to a patient as an answer to the question 'How important is this to me?'.

If we return to examination of the the data from Doll's nickel refinery study, we see that the next step was to calculate the death rate from lung cancer in those workers who had begun work in the refinery **after** 1925. The result is shown in Table 5.3.

Table 5.3 Age-standardised death rates in nickel workers in a South Wales refinery employed before and after 1925.[1]

Exposure history	Lung cancer death rate per 1000 PYR
Employed before 1925	17.94
Employed after 1925	1.96

We have seen that the lung cancer rate in those men first employed before 1925 was 17.94 per 1 000 PYR; the rate in those men employed after 1925 was only 1.96. Subtracting one rate from the other we have an attributable risk.

Attributable Risk = (17.94 − 1.96) per 1000 PYR = 15.98 per 1000 PYR.

This suggests that engineering changes made in the refinery processes in about 1925 effectively removed the lung cancer hazard. The benefit of these actions can be expressed as 15.98 deaths prevented for each 1 000 PYR worked in the refinery. Relative risk gives us a measure of the strength of an association; attributable risk gives us a way of estimating the cost benefits of a preventive programme.

OTHER FACTORS INFLUENCING PROGNOSIS

Rose made the following comment on the relevance of epidemiology to clinical practice: 'In teaching epidemiology to medical students, I have often encouraged them to consider the question: "why did this patient get this disease at this time?"'[4]

There are a number of factors that influence the risk that an individual, exposed to a potentially harmful agent, will actually be harmed. For example, a certain level of blood pressure may be more dangerous in a smoker or someone with a high plasma cholesterol. There are a number of other factors that will influence how a particular individual or patient will progress. These are related either to the characteristics of the disease or to the characteristics of the individual. For example, patients referred to hospital because of a disease tend to have it in a more severe form than those managed in general practice. If a doctor were to give advice about disease risk or prognosis based on hospital experience alone, then that advice would be unlikely to be accurate.

Some of the factors which might influence the outcome of an illness include:

Who you are: age, sex, social class, ethnic background;
Other characteristics: medical history, personal behaviour (smoking, homosexuality), presence of other disease;
Where you are: hospital, general practice, screening program;
Level of disease: stage to which disease has progressed;
Form of treatment: advice, drug therapy, surgery.

CAUSE AND EFFECT
....

The basis of the practice of preventive medicine lies in an understanding of the natural history of a disease and, in particular, in knowledge of its cause or causes. Attribution of cause is fairly simple at one level, for example there is not much discussion as to the cause of tuberculosis—although this has not always been the case. At another level, the cause of coronary heart disease is quite complex. In public health generally, deciding that some factor is a cause of a common disease can lead to widespread economic consequences—the swing from butter to margarine had a considerable effect on the livelihood of dairy farmers—an effect that needs to be balanced against health gains. A most costly exercise in preventive medicine is the removal of lead from petrol. In short, correct attribution of cause is an important aspect of the practice of medicine in its broader and advisory sense.

Figure 5.2 shows the simplest form of a causal relationship; in this case, C is necessary for disease E to occur. Infection by the mycobacterium is a necessary condition for tuberculosis to occur, though whether the disease actually manifests itself depends upon a large number of host factors, such as immune state, nutrition and age. In other words, whilst the presence of the mycobacterium is necessary, this in itself is not sufficient to produce the disease.

41

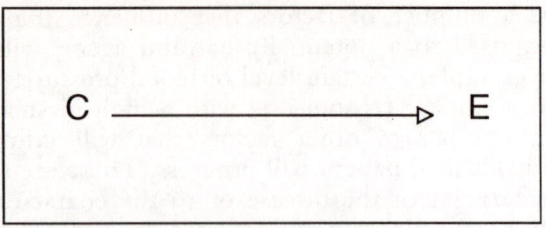

Figure 5.2 *C is necessary for E to occur.*

Non-causal associations are found not infrequently; one such form of association is shown in Figure 5.3.

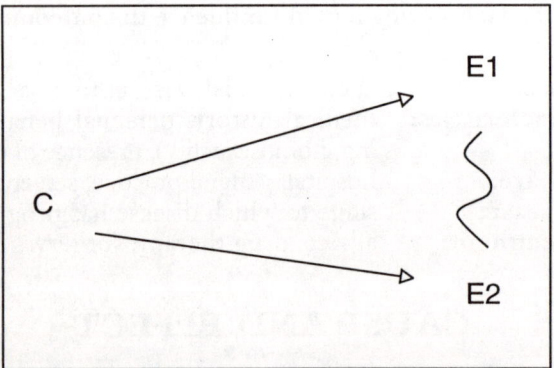

Figure 5.3 *E1 and E2 have a non-causal association.*

In Figure 5.3 the common factor C causes both E1 and E2 and it is therefore evident that E1 and E2 will often be found together. This association is non-causal in that E1 does not cause E2 (or vice versa). One would expect chronic bronchitis and bladder cancer to occur together in the same person more often than chance alone would dictate, not because one causes the other but rather because smoking is a common causal factor.

A very common situation is that in which the disease E has a number of causes, illustrated below in Figure 5.4. For example, exposure to asbestos (C1) is a cause of lung cancer (E) but so is cigarette smoking (C2). Lung cancer, of course, may occur in the absence of either.

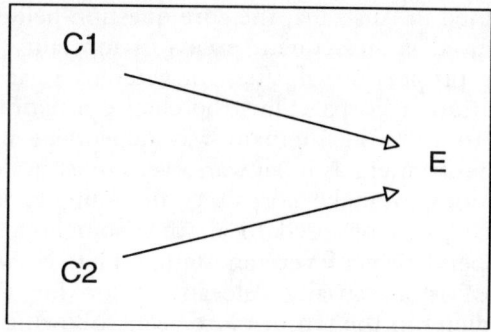

Figure 5.4 *C1 and C2 are each causes of E.*

If one were studying a possible relationship between exposure to asbestos and development of lung cancer, a reasonable plan would be to compare the incidence of lung cancer in a group of men who had worked with asbestos, with that found in a similar group of men who had never experienced asbestos exposure. If by chance, the non-exposed men were all heavy cigarette smokers and the exposed men were all non-smokers, then a comparison between the two asbestos groups would seriously underestimate the true risk of asbestos exposure because of imbalance between the two groups with respect to smoking. In technical terms the comparison is said to be 'confounded', and the smoking habits of the men would be called a 'confounding variable'.

A confounding variable (F) distorts the association between a causal factor and the effect by being associated with the causal factor and by being itself another cause of the effect, as illustrated in Figure 5.5.

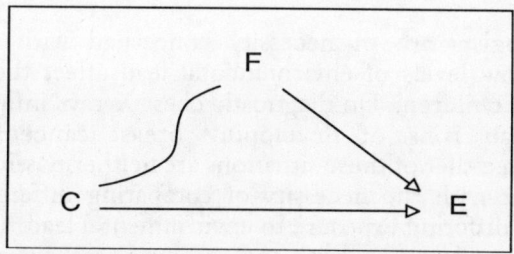

Figure 5.5 *C is a cause of E. F is associated with C, and is itself a cause of E. F is a confounding variable.*

An interesting 'real world' example of such a confounding variable occurred in the study of mortality in Australian Vietnam veterans over the years following the end of that conflict.[2] The essential comparison was between national servicemen who had served in Vietnam and those who had remained in Australia, the core question being whether such service (C) 'caused' a subsequent excess of mortality (E). Table 5.4 shows that the proportion of Vietnam veterans varied considerably between the different corps. Thus the chance a national serviceman had of going to fight in Vietnam was dependent upon his corps designation; infantrymen, as in all wars, were most in demand.

In itself this does not make 'corps' a confounding variable (F), unless being in one corps as opposed to another somehow influenced the outcome, independently of veteran status. That is, we need to ask whether 'corps' is a causally relevant factor for the outcome— probability of dying in the ten or more years following the end of the war. Table 5.4 shows that the mortality rates among non-veterans of the different corps were different. Thus in any comparison of Vietnam veterans with non-veterans like must be compared with like—infantry with infantry, engineers with engineers and so forth.

Table 5.4 Proportion of veterans by Army Corps. All cause mortality, over period of follow-up per 10 000 among non-veterans.

Corps	*Proportion of veterans within corps grouping (%)*	*Mortality rate per 10^4 (non-veterans)*
Infantry	61	13.0
Engineers	52	5.7
Armour and artillery	48	11.1
Minor field presence	28	5.6
Non-field corps	27	9.0

Epidemiologists are of necessity concerned with observational studies. Do low levels of environmental lead affect the growth and maturation of children? Do diagnostic chest X-rays influence the risk that a woman runs of developing breast cancer? Controlled experiments in either of these situations are neither possible nor ethical so we are left with the necessity of comparing different groups of children with differing exposure to environmental lead, and examining the past history of women (with and without breast cancer).

When assessing whether some observed association is causal, one can do worse than follow Sir Austin Bradford Hill's criteria for causation in observational studies.[5]

1. Strength of association
2. Consistency
3. Time relationships
4. Biological gradient

5. Biological plausibility
6. Coherence of the evidence
7. Experiment
8. Analogy

As Hill himself noted, none of these criteria is indispensable but together they form a useful guide to establishing causation in the absence of rigorous experimentation. A ninth criterion was specificity, that is the requirement that a cause produces one and only one effect, but today this is regarded as inconsistent with current biological knowledge.

ASSESSING CAUSATION
....

1. Strength of the association
Workers exposed to benzene are 5–25 times more likely to develop leukaemia than are people not so exposed. This is a reasonably strong association and as a consequence is likely to represent a causal relationship. By way of contrast, the risk leather workers run of developing bladder cancer is only 1.5 times that experienced by other workers and, as a consequence, one is far less sure of the relationship being causal.

2. Consistency
'One swallow doesn't make a summer'—has the observation been made in different places, different circumstances and times, and by different persons? The relationships between cigarette smoking and lung cancer, exposure to asbestos and mesothelioma, and blood cholesterol levels and coronary heart disease, are all examples where findings have been consistent in different countries, at different times, and between different research teams.

3. Appropriate time relationships
In general, of course, a cause must precede an effect. This issue is not always as obvious as you might think. If children who consume lead from the soil as babies are later shown to have an IQ deficit, did the lead consumption cause the deficit, or did their lower IQ (as babies) cause them to be 'dirt eaters'?

Cancer usually has a long latent period and if, for example, an association was found between a chemical exposure and a cancer and there was a very short time period between the events, one should be cautious about accepting this as a causal relationship.

4. Biological gradient

The presence of a biological gradient, or 'dose-response curve' is a powerful argument for an association being causal. The causal nature of the relationship between smoking and lung cancer is much strengthened by the step-wise increase in incidence of cancer with increasing number of cigarettes smoked.

5. Biological plausibility

What is biologically plausible depends, of course, on the biological knowledge of the day. Whilst it is pleasing to have such support, it is worth remembering the prize essay written in the 19th century which stated '... it would be ridiculous for the stranger who passed the night in the steerage of an emigrant ship to ascribe the typhus, which he contracted, to the vermin with which bodies of the sick might be infested ...'.

6. Coherence of the evidence

To quote Bradford Hill once more, 'the cause and effect interpretation of our data should not seriously conflict with the generally known facts of the natural history and biology of the disease'. That is to say, the epidemiological findings should fit in with observations from other disciplines.

7. Experiment

Sometimes 'experimental' findings are available. Suppose that previous evidence has led to the introduction of a preventive programme. Then if the effect is abolished or diminished by removing the supposed cause, this is probably the most powerful argument linking cause and effect. Support from animal experimentation is very important. Occasionally data arise from human 'natural experiments', such as occurred in 1954 with an intense period of fog in London. Very closely associated in time was a major increase in mortality not only from chest diseases, as would have been expected, but also from other causes.

8. Analogy

It would seem reasonable to ascribe causation if a similar mechanism has been shown to operate for another condition. Our knowledge of the effects of rubella in pregnancy, for example, might make us more willing to accept weaker but analogous findings concerning exposure to similar agents in pregnant women.

RISK FACTORS AND POPULATIONS
·······

Risk factors for disease are distributed throughout populations. Those measured on a continuous scale often follow a 'normal' or 'bell-shaped' curve. As a consequence, it should be possible to distinguish a group of people at the high end of the distribution who may be characterised as high risk and thus to concentrate scarce preventive health resources on them. Whilst this concept, known as the 'high risk strategy', makes sense it does contain a paradox well shown in Table 5.5 which has been taken from Rose.[6]

Down syndrome is a birth defect characterised by severe intellectual disability and abnormalities in one or more organs. The major risk factor is known to be increasing maternal age and, as shown in the table, the relationship is strong with the risk increasing from 0.4 per 1000 births in younger women to 8.1 in the oldest group. The paradox is that if women over 45 were to be prevented from having children, the reduction in the number of babies born with Down syndrome would be trivial. The same situation is true of coronary heart disease where risk is defined not simply by age but by the presence or degree of a large number of personal or behavioural characteristics known as 'risk factors'. Because heart attacks are so common, most of them occur in people properly designated as 'low risk'. This is another illustration of the difference between relative and attributable measures of risk.

Table 5.5 Maternal age and Down syndrome, England and Wales 1979–85.[6]

Maternal age	Birth prevalence of Down syndrome per 1 000 births	% all births by maternal age group	% Down syndrome occurring in this group
Under 20	0.4	9	5
20–24	0.4	30	17
25–29	0.5	34	25
30–34	1.0	19	27
35–39	2.2	6	18
40–44	5.1	1	7
45 +	8.1	0.1	1
All ages	0.7	100	100

Figure 5.6 comes from a survey of 909 men living in the Hunter Valley[7] and shows the distribution of alcohol consumption on 'a day when you drink alcohol'; non-drinkers are labelled 'nil'. A worthwhile

goal for health promotion would be to have nobody in the population at the highest end of the distribution, say over nine drinks a day, and to have reduced the number of men drinking five or more drinks a day. One approach would be to use the high risk strategy mentioned above and here we might recall the heavy drinkers for intensive group or one-on-one counselling. An alternative strategy depends on a population view of health. It has now been well established that, when a number of different populations are studied, the level of the mean or average drinking pattern is strongly related to the proportion of heavy drinkers in that population.[8] It follows that a relatively small reduction in the mean number of drinks per day characterising a population would shift the entire distribution downwards, with a quite substantial reduction in the number of high risk drinkers in that population.[6]

The high risk strategy is a direct development from experience with clinical patient care and for this reason appeals to health professionals. Because the population approach calls for skills honed in political activism, advertising, and marketing, there is little room for those whose view is totally encompassed by traditional clinical skills. Occasionally these differing views result in unhelpful conflict in the eternal chase for the dollar but in the best of all possible worlds both the high risk and the population strategies would be used to reduce risk in a population.

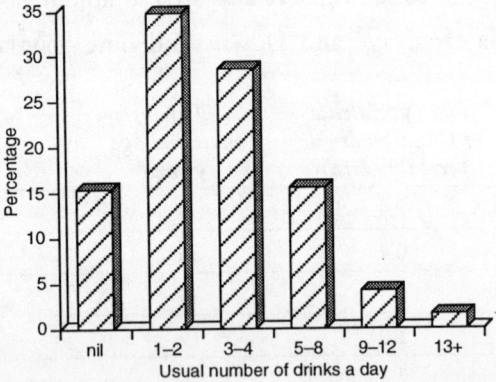

Figure 5.6 *Usual number of alcoholic drinks on a day when alcohol is consumed, for men living in the Hunter Valley.*[7]

EXERCISES

Exercise 5.1

Coronary heart disease (CHD) is of multifactorial cause, the risk factors including tobacco smoking, diet and serum cholesterol, high blood pressure, sedentary lifestyle and diabetes. A screening examination was carried out on the population of a large industrial complex comprising 8 398 men and information was obtained on the above risk factors.[9] From these a composite score was developed and the top 15% of the distribution were regarded as those at greatest risk. The number of men developing a heart attack over the next five years, by original risk category, is shown in Table 5.6.

1. Do you think that the risk score was effective in categorising men at high risk of heart attack? Explain your answer.
2. How much improvement in the 'heart health' of the workforce, as measured by the occurrence of heart attacks, do you think would be achieved by a health counselling programme targeting only the identified high risk men?
3. Do you think that the information from the screening programme would be of value to the men concerned and could there be any unwanted 'side effects' of such activity?

Table 5.6 Risk of a fatal or non-fatal myocardial infarction by risk score in 8 398 men at a large individual complex.

Risk category	No. of men	No. of heart attacks
High (top 15%)	1 283	119
Not high (85%)	7 115	248
Total	8 398	367

Exercise 5.2

The medical history of 18 228 men was followed for five years following a cardiovascular screening examination which included an electrocardiogram (ECG) and a standard questionnaire on angina. Table 5.7 shows the coronary heart disease mortality of the group according to the findings at the initial examination.[8] Note that 'angina' is chest pain characteristically of heart origin and an 'ischaemic ECG' is an electrocardiogram whose features indicate the presence of coronary heart disease.

Table 5.7 The number of men in each category at time of screening examination and the number who died of CHD over the next five years.

On entry	No. of men	Deaths from CHD
1 No angina, no ischaemic ECG	15 431	139
2 Angina only	1 654	55
3 Ischaemic ECG only	889	38
4 Angina and ischaemic ECG	254	42
Total	*18 228*	*274*

For each of the groups 2 to 4 above calculate the relative and attributable risks of dying of CHD within five years.

Exercise 5.3

In a population of 100 000, 30% were current cigarette smokers and Table 5.8 shows the number of lung cancers expected to occur over a year's observation. The rates of occurrence of lung cancer are taken from Doll and Hill's study of British doctors.[10]

Table 5.8 Expected incidence and number of lung cancers in a population

	No.	Incidence of lung cancer	'Expected' cancers
Smokers	30 000	7.6 per 10 000 per year	22.8
Non-smokers	70 000	0.9 per 10 000 per year	6.3

If nobody smoked in this population, the expected number of cancers would have been nine (from the rate in non-smokers of 0.9 per 10^5 per year). Thus, of the 29 cancers that actually occurred, 20 may be attributed to smoking, which is 69%. This is sometimes known as the 'population attributable risk per cent'.

Calculate the percentage of lung cancers that could be attributed to cigarette smoking if:
1. 15% of a population smoked.
2. 55% of a population smoked.

ANSWERS

Exercise 5.1

1. Quite effective. The top 15% contain one third of the heart attacks (119/367) and as a way of categorising high risk the score worked quite well.

2. Not as much as one would have liked to think. Suppose that through effective health counselling the occurrence rate of heart attacks in the high risk group could be halved. This would mean a reduction in attack rate from 8.7 per thousand per year to 7.3 per thousand per year (367/8 398 to 307/8 398 and divide by five to get an annual rate).

3. It would certainly encourage those men labelled 'high risk' to follow appropriate advice, such as stopping smoking, dietary change and taking exercise. The possible side effects might include engendering fear and 'medicalising' healthy people. It also might not be wise for the non-high risk men to think that they do not need any adjustment to their lifestyle.

Exercise 5.2

1. (reference group):
   5 year risk = 139/15431 = 9.01 per 1000
2. (angina only):
   5 year risk = 55/1654 = 33.25 per 1000
   relative risk = 33.25/9.01 = 3.7
   attributable risk = 33.25 - 9.01 = 24.24 per 1000
3. (ischaemic ECG only):
   5 year risk = 38/889 = 42.74 per 1000
   relative risk = 42.74/9.01 = 4.7
   attributable risk = 42.74 - 9.01 = 33.73 per 1000
4. (angina + ischaemic ECG):
   5 year risk = 42/254 = 165.35 per 1000
   relative risk = 165.35/9.01 = 18.4
   attributable risk = 165.35 - 9.01 = 156.34 per 1000

Note that these calculations have used risks rather than rates since the data to calculate rates were not given.

Exercise 5.3

In general, the population attributable risk percentage depends on the proportion of the population exposed.

If the whole population of 100 000 were non-smokers, we would expect 9.0 lung cancers on average.

Table 5.9 Calculations for the population attributable risk.

	Population 1 (15% smokers)		Population 2 (55% smokers)	
	Number	*Number of expected lung cancers*	*Number*	*Number of expected lung cancers*
Smokers	15 000	11.4	55 000	41.8
Non-smokers	85 000	7.7	45 000	4.1
Total	*100 000*	*19.1*	*100 000*	*45.9*
Excess due to smoking		10.1		36.9
Population attributable risk %		53		80

CHAPTER SIX

INTRODUCTION TO RESEARCH: SURVEYS OR CROSS-SECTIONAL STUDIES

❧

Research in the health sciences involves finding out more about the world in which we live and in particular how we, its inhabitants, relate to the environment in which we find ourselves. First of all we need to decide what it is that we wish to explore and it is helpful to express this thought in the form of an hypothesis. Last[1] defines an hypothesis as a 'supposition, arrived at from observation or reflection, that leads to refutable predictions'. In other words, an hypothesis is in the first place a statement of how somebody thinks the world is. Consider two such statements:

> Good dogs go to heaven.
> The moon is made of green cheese.

Each of these statements may be believed by a person, but an important difference is that only the second can be tested empirically as to its truth or falsehood. That is to say, observations can be made and, by careful consideration, a judgement can be made as to how likely the belief is to be true.

What then must an hypothesis contain? The first requirement—and many would say the only requirement—is a statement that is capable of being refuted. Possibly the most famous hypothesis was formulated as follows:

> Every body continues in its state of rest, or of uniform motion
> in a straight line, unless it is compelled to change that state by
> forces acting on it.

Newton evidently felt no need to specify the circumstances under which his belief would hold, and he expressed no interest in the methods fellow scientists might use in their attempts to refute or falsify his hypothesis. Nevertheless, it is quite possible to test by experiment whether this statement is in fact true and, what is more, such testing is carried out in high school physics laboratories.

There are other statements which relate to ourselves and the world in which we live, and one such reads as follows:[2]

> …King Oedipus, who slew his father Laius and wedded his
> mother Jocasta, is nothing more or less than a wish-fulfilment—
> the fulfilment of the wish of our childhood.
> But we, more fortunate than he, in so far as we have not
> become psychoneurotics, have since our childhood succeeded
> in withdrawing our sexual impulses from our mothers, and in
> forgetting our jealousy of our fathers…

It is doubtful whether it ever crossed Sigmund Freud's mind that any of his opinions could be wrong, certainly there is no way of testing them. This absence of any testable component, whilst it has nothing to do with the truth or otherwise of Freudian psychology, does mean that the latter cannot be classified as a science.

Hypotheses concerned with humans and their behaviour usually need to be related to times, places, and other specifics, much more than do hypotheses which are concerned with the physical world. Consider the following:

> An increased body burden of lead is associated with impaired
> intellectual functioning.

This hypothesis is not concerned with exactly how the body burden of lead will be measured, nor with the manner in which intellectual functioning will be assessed. However, unlike the situation that presumably holds in physics, in applied biological science it is usually necessary to state the framework within which the hypothesis is expected to hold; Miettinen[3] refers to this framework as the 'domain of the relationship'. The reason is that in biology the postulated effect is often modified by other characteristics of the subjects. In the case of lead and intellectual functioning, age is an obvious modifier and children are much more susceptible to the effects of lead on the central nervous system than are adults. So the above hypothesis might be narrowed to:

> In children an increased body burden of lead is associated with
> impaired intellectual functioning.

In summary, the essential kernel contained in an hypothesis is a statement to which empirical data can be applied in order to refute it, if possible.

THE SURVEY
·······

Of the various research strategies available to test an epidemiological hypothesis, the commonest by far is the survey. The main feature of the survey is that people provide information at a point in time and for this reason surveys are also known as prevalence or cross-sectional studies. Sometimes a whole population is surveyed—'what do the residents of a housing estate think of a proposed freeway?'—but it is more usual for a sample to be taken. For proper interpretation of the results, the sample needs to be 'representative' of a larger population and to have been drawn in an unbiased manner, preferably by random sampling. Figure 6.1 is a schematic representation of the 'hierarchy of populations' with which we are concerned in sample surveys.

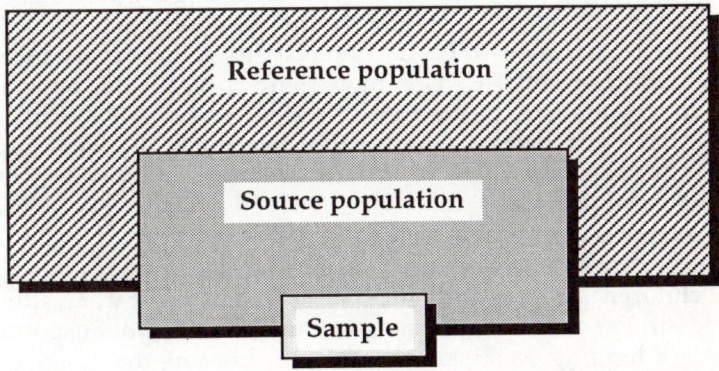

Figure 6.1 *Sample, source population, and reference population.*

Sample
These are the actual people from whom information is obtained. They are the sample whose names have been drawn, for example, from the electoral roll. Not everyone is going to consent to take part and thus the sample really consists of the responders, those people who attend the survey or complete the questionnaire.

Source population
This is the population with which the study is directly concerned. A sample could be drawn from school lists representing all adolescents in the Hunter Valley, and then the source population would be all those teenagers. Unlike the sample, the source population is not restricted to those who actually completed the questionnaire.

Reference population

This is an abstract concept of the people about whom the researcher wishes to make a statement. In the example above the reference population might be all adolescents or perhaps all adolescents in Australia.

When the results of the survey are to be interpreted, it is necessary to consider whether the sample provides a reasonable estimate of circumstances holding in firstly the source population and, if so, in the reference population. The response rate to the survey is critical in making this judgement, as is knowledge of the degree of homogeneity of the populations. From a carefully designed survey, quantitative inferences can be made from the sample to the source population. Problems arise and mistakes are made when inferences about the reference population are made from data collected in the sample. For example, the behaviour of a rural sample of adolescents is likely to provide little guidance when the interest lies in teenagers living in Sydney's western suburbs. Common sense is invaluable in making these judgements and, in the case of the teenagers above, it is likely that the rates of repair of bone fractures are much the same because this rate probably has little to do with cultural differences between different social groups.

The survey is at its best when used to estimate a current reality, such as the prevalence of self-reported cigarette smoking in Hunter Valley school children[4] as shown in Figure 6.2. It is at its worst when attempts are made to use the survey to suggest causal links—'does exposure to fluorescent lighting cause skin cancer?'. In choosing the design of the survey the question to be asked must be appropriate to the method and its limitations; in Figure 6.2, however, the answers have been given to an entirely appropriate question. Similarly questions in other populations might be as follows.

What is the prevalence of high blood pressure in a country town?
What is the prevalence of chronic cough in the Latrobe Valley?
What is the exact job description of workers in a chemical factory?

These are all appropriate questions because they deal with factual information, common conditions, and they relate to the here and now.

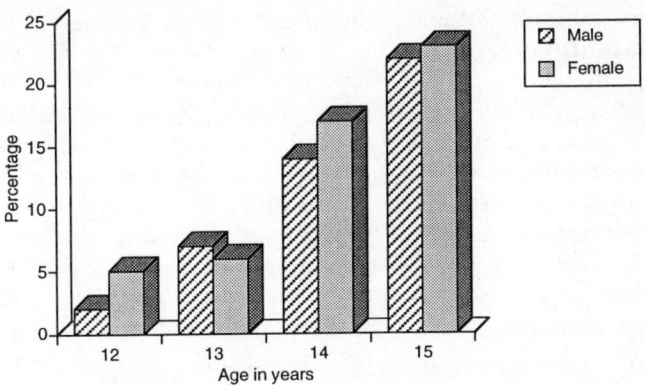

Figure 6.2 *Percentage of children aged 12–15 in a Hunter Valley survey who reported having smoked in the last week.*[4]

Where a causal association is being sought by use of a survey, the presumed cause or 'risk factor' needs to be not only common but strongly related to the effect. In another Hunter Valley survey,[5] men and women were asked whether they agreed or disagreed with the statement 'there is really no way I can solve the problems I have'. The sense of powerlessness implied by agreement with this statement is not uncommon in our society and this is clearly shown in Table 6.1. It will surprise few that an association with gender is present with women more likely to feel powerless to change their lives.

Table 6.1 Responses, by gender, to the statement 'there is really no way I can solve the problems I have'.

	Strongly agree	*Agree*	*Not sure*	*Disagree*	*Strongly disagree*	
Male	8	44	26	185	109	372
	(2.1%)	(11.8%)	(7.0%)	(49.7%)	(29.4%)	(100%)
Female	18	63	27	176	80	364
	(4.9%)	(17.3%)	(7.4%)	(48.4%)	(22.0%)	(100%)
All	*26*	*107*	*53*	*361*	*189*	*736*

The great weakness of the cross-sectional survey is that it does not have a time dimension built into it. In assessing whether a relationship is truly causal, time relationships are most important—a cause must come before an effect. Consider a survey in which alcohol consumption and occupational stress were measured. If excessive consumption were found to be associated with high stress levels at work, we could not conclude from the survey alone whether the stress led to the drinking pattern, or the other way around, or indeed whether both were caused by some third factor.

The other problem with cross-sectional surveys, particularly in the health sciences, is that the only people who can be asked questions or examined are those who are available to be asked—the 'survivor' problem or bias. Consider a survey in which all motorcyclists and every tenth car driver on a freeway were stopped and asked whether over the last 12 months they had been in a serious road accident. Suppose further that the accident rate among car drivers was found to be twice that of motorcyclists. There are several possible conclusions including:

1. Cars are more dangerous than motorcycles.
2. Serious road accidents are more likely to kill motorcyclists than car drivers.
3. After a serious accident, motorcyclists tend to give up riding motorcycles in favour of driving a car.

Each conclusion is logically possible because, if no. 2 or 3 is correct, there is a selection bias operating which tends to remove motorcyclists who have had serious accidents from future participation in surveys. Selection biases can be more subtle. It has been frequently stated that migraine is associated with intelligence and high social class, firstly by Fothergill in 1784, quoted by Waters,[6] who pronounced that 'sick headache' was found mostly in the 'middle and upper ranks of life'. *Harrison's Principles of Internal Medicine*,[7] as recently as 20 years ago, reiterated that 'migraine patients tend to be intelligent'. Estlin Waters, following a community survey of migraine,[6] classified migraine sufferers both by social class and by their willingness to consult a doctor. He showed that, of migraine sufferers, 81% of those from the professional and executive classes would usually see a doctor, compared with only 63% of those who were semi-skilled or unskilled labourers. Thus it would seem that while the patients doctors see with migraine are of higher social class, distribution of migraine in the community extends across all social classes. This is an example of selection bias where doctors are seeing a self-selected group of individuals.

RESPONSE RATES

Any teacher surveying a class knows perfectly well that the bright-eyed children who sit in the front row are different from the layabouts skulking up the back. When a question is asked, those children with the hands up shouting 'Miss, Miss, Miss...' could by no stretch of the imagination be regarded as a random sample of the class.

In a survey, those people who volunteer to answer the questions are also very likely to be systematically different from those who refuse to cooperate. The problem is one of external validity and for inferences from a sample to a larger population to be made it is absolutely essential that the response rate be quite high. In 'health' surveys, younger people are generally under-represented. When mass chest X-ray surveys were being carried out those who did not attend were shown repeatedly to have more likelihood of having tuberculosis than those who did attend. In reports of surveys the response rate must be very critically examined. A survey should be carried out in a defined population and the response rate is the ratio of those who responded to those who could have responded.

$$\text{Response rate} = \frac{\text{number of people who responded}}{\text{number who could have responded}}$$

In a 1985 study in Melbourne,[8] researchers attempted to interview men who had been convicted 10 years earlier of a drink-driving offence. Two-thirds of the study population were interviewed, but one-third had either moved interstate or overseas, refused to be interviewed, or just could not be found. Table 6.2 shows the number of alcohol-related offences for which the interviewed and non-interviewed men had been convicted during those 10 years. The difference is quite marked and illustrates what is known as 'non-responder bias'.

Table 6.2 Alcohol-related convictions in responders and non-responders.

	Number of alcohol-related offences			
	0	1	2	3 +
Interviewed	71%	14%	8%	7%
Not interviewed	60%	10%	14%	16%

The situation with regard to response rates is summarised in Figure 6.3. A response rate of over 80% indicates good preparation and one can be reasonably confident in extrapolating the results to similar populations. With the response rate between 60% and 80% more work needs to be done and the lower the response rate the more energetic the research team is going to have to be in encouraging the non-responders and at least finding out as much as possible about them in socio-demographic terms. After all attempts to increase the response to something above 60% have failed, there is serious cause for concern about possible response bias.

In a recent comment on a survey, whose response rate was 47%, a leader of the profession concerned commented in the newspapers that 'for this type of (mailed) survey the response rate was quite good'. In fact, Figure 6.3 clearly labels the survey in question as problematic. Getting a high response rate is not easy and demands a lot of preparation and patience.

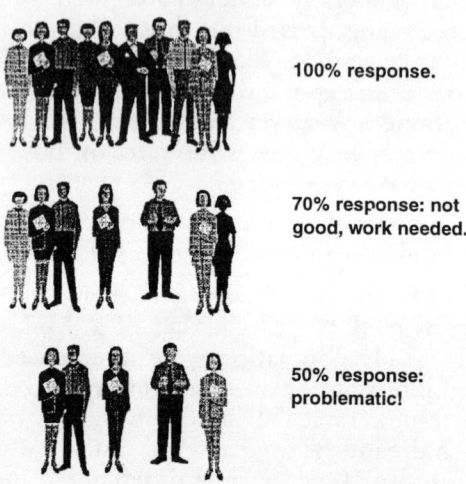

100% response.

70% response: not good, work needed.

50% response: problematic!

Figure 6.3 *Survey response rates and their meaning.*

VALIDITY

In Figure 6.1 the relationship between sample surveys and higher order populations was described. The extent to which such extrapolation is reasonable is known as the external validity of the survey and depends largely on selection of study populations and sampling techniques. On the other hand, the internal validity of a survey, or indeed any similar study, is dependent upon the validity of each component of the collected data. A useful and general definition of validity is that of Last.[1]

> An expression of the degree to which a measurement measures what it purports to measure.

When considering tests or questions the term 'criterion validity' is often used and Last defines this as:

> The extent to which the measurement correlates with an external criterion of the phenomenon under study.

This may be paraphrased into an assessment of the degree to which a question or test measures what we think it is measuring. When physiological tests, such as blood pressure or pulmonary function, are being made we are usually only able to measure a surrogate of the real thing. For example, we use a sphygmomanometer reading in lieu of a direct measure of intra-arterial blood pressure. In terms of a reported behaviour, such as alcohol consumption or drug taking, we ask a question and then need to be able to assess the likelihood that our subjects are telling the truth. To have confidence in the validity of a statement or measurement some objective standard is needed, at least on a sample. The latter is often referred to as a 'gold standard' but in practice the word bronze is that which springs more readily to mind!

In a survey where the interest was in analgesic consumption, the question concerning aspirin and paracetamol taking was checked against a drug analysis of urine samples.[9] Where all else fails an indirect form of validation can be helpful as when the alcohol consumption patterns of a workforce were found to be very similar to those reported from a union survey in the same Australian State.[10]

Validation is difficult but, where the data are important, an attempt must be made to 'get some kind of handle on it'.

EXERCISES

Exercise 6.1

Possibly the most disastrously inaccurate survey of all time was carried out by the American magazine *Literary Digest* before the 1936 United States Presidential election. It is also usually held to be the largest survey of all time. This was in a depression year and the Republican candidate, Alfred M. Landon, was running against the Democrat incumbent, Franklin D. Roosevelt. The magazine sent out a questionnaire to each of its subscribers and to a collection of people randomly selected from telephone directories across the nation. The final sample consisted of 2.4 million people and, from their replies, the magazine was able to predict a landslide victory for Landon—it predicted that his vote would be 57%. In the event, the election proved almost a total victory for Roosevelt who carried all but two States and Landon's vote was 38%. (Incidentally, the magazine went into liquidation within six months of the survey.)

1. Why do you think that this survey produced results so at variance with reality?
2. The magazine editors obviously thought that a sample size of 2.4 million people lent enormous credibility to the results. Do you agree, and if not, why not?

3. If the sample question 'how did you vote last time?' had been asked as well as 'who are you going to vote for?' do you think that the magazine would have gone ahead and published its predictions?
4. George Gallup was setting up his survey organisation at this time. Using 50 000 people (2.1% of the size of the *Digest*'s sample) he correctly predicted the Roosevelt victory. How do you think he obtained his sample?

Exercise 6.2

Once upon a time in a far away Kingdom many years ago the media and people were becoming very agitated about increasing urban air pollution from industrialisation. The King's response was to have a random sample survey of the city's population carried out every five years, in order to examine them for chest disease and to measure their lung function. Deterioration over time would thus indicate increasing pollution in the city. This plan was tried out, and over a 20 year period the urban pollution really did seem to get much worse but the random samples of the city population showed no change in the proportion of people with chest disease (which in fact was quite low), nor was there any appreciable change in lung function, nor any change in the cigarette smoking habits of the people. 'There' said the King 'there is no pollution and it is all in your imagination'. The population at this remark revolted and, bringing the King before the People's Court, accused him of quoting biased statistics. He, of course, lost his head. What was the most likely source of the bias?

ANSWERS

Exercise 6.1

1. In the depression year of 1936 only those reasonably well off and employed would be likely to have a telephone, the possession of which in any case had not penetrated society to anything like its modern extent. Of these people, those who would read and subscribe to a magazine called *Literary Digest* are an even more select population. The sample could have had no external validity as a guide to the views held by all voting Americans, principally because of the bias towards the conservative end of the political spectrum. Furthermore, the response rate for the survey was poor at 24% as the *Digest* had actually sought the views of 10 million voters!
2. There is little argument that 2.4 million people is a staggeringly large sample size. Nevertheless, the reliability of a sample in terms of its probable relationship to the 'true' population parameter increases not by the number of subjects in the sample but in terms

of the square root of that number. Thus a four-fold increase in sample size only doubles the reliability, a one-hundred fold expansion increases it by ten. For this reason, when interpreting the value of a survey, the number of subjects in the sample is of far less importance than are considerations of how much care was taken in its construction so that it might be reasonably representative of the source and reference populations from which it was drawn. The *Digest*'s problem lay not in sample size but in the biased nature of that sample.

3. A question on previous voting performance would have signalled very clearly the non-representativeness of the sample and, hopefully, would have acted as a red light to the pollsters!

4. Once more it is not the size of the sample that is of the most importance in a survey, rather it is how representative that sample is of some reference population. Gallup used a sampling method that ensured that the distributions of major features of the sample were the same as those in the population.

Exercise 6.2

Once more it is a case of selective recruitment to a survey or series of surveys. As soon as people start to cough and splutter in the mornings they pack up and take themselves, and their families, to healthier climates. Their houses are bought, and their jobs filled, by people down from the country. This means that the only people available to become members of the random samples are the fresh-faced (and fresh-chested) country boys and girls, those people who have not yet got chest disease, and those who are for some reason less susceptible to chest disease.

Consideration of how people become members of a particular population, and remain members of it, is very important in studies carried out in any closed population, such as a workforce. Perhaps entry is preceded by a rigorous pre-employment medical; perhaps people get discharged if they become ill; perhaps they can stay on 'forever' as some people seem to be able to do in certain jobs. In other words, before embarking on a survey in an industrial population we need to know about managerial and personnel practices.

CHAPTER SEVEN

LONGITUDINAL STUDIES

Surveys, or cross-sectional studies, suffer from the inherent defect that they contain no time component. Not only are incidence measures impossible but confusion can occur in the disentangling of cause–effect relationships: 'which came first, the chicken or the egg?'

In longitudinal or prospective studies, subjects are defined not in terms of having or not having a particular disease but rather in terms of exposure to a possible cause of that disease. Thus a prospective study, the purpose of which was to investigate alcohol consumption as a cause of oesophageal cancer, would begin by defining a population which could be characterised on varying degrees of alcohol consumption. This is in contrast to a case–control study where the population would be defined on the presence or absence of the cancer. Having defined the exposure profile of the population, it is then followed over time, and relevant health outcomes are recorded.

COHORT STUDIES

Prospective studies are often termed cohort studies because a group of people, say, workers at a factory at a particular time, are followed in terms of their health experience over many years. A cohort was a Roman military formation and, like most military formations, presumably spent a lot of time on route marches. In epidemiology the term denotes a body of people with some common experience who 'march together', not along a Roman road but rather through time.

Some general concepts of longitudinal data and their interpretation follow, including a discussion of planned longitudinal studies.

Birth Cohorts

The members of a cohort share a common experience and one such experience is that of being born during the same calendar period, or interval of time—a cohort defined in these terms is known as a birth cohort.

Over the last 50 years the change in lung cancer mortality in Australian men has been remarkable. The age-specific rates have increased in each adult age group until more recently, when a plateau has been observed. Such an analysis, whilst indicating quite clearly that there is a problem, does not in itself generate any hypotheses as to possible causes or indicate possible lines of research. Another form of analysis of mortality data is known as cohort analysis. Here, instead of studying changes in age-specific rates at successive points in calendar time, the mortality experience of successive birth cohorts as they pass through different age groups is examined. In the following example, a cohort analysis is carried out on the Australian mortality data from lung cancer in men.

Table 7.1 shows death rates from lung cancer and each entry is the average of the relevant age-specific rate over the five years of the particular calendar period. Thus the men contributing to the rate for age 35–39, calendar period 1950–54, were all born in the years 1911–19. In this way we can form cohorts that share a median year of birth, in this case 1915. The table shows the death rates of three cohorts with median years of birth 1915, 1905 and 1895, respectively. The death rates of these cohorts as they age are represented along the diagonals. The data are shown graphically in Figure 7.1 and this is perhaps the easiest way to see the pattern emerging.

In a classic cohort analysis of deaths in Britain in the earlier half of this century Case[1] showed each generation to have a higher death rate from lung cancer at all ages than the generation which preceded it. This indicated that the cause of the change was some factor associated with being a member of one birth cohort as opposed to another, probably a lifestyle difference. As it happened, the time patterns of tobacco smoking prevalence coincided neatly with the changes in lung cancer. In the Australian data for the cohorts born around 1895 and 1905 (page 66) this pattern is repeated with higher lung cancer mortality in the more recent cohort at every age. However, in the most recent cohort, those men born around 1915, the pattern changes when they arrive in their seventies (in the 1980s) and the death rate falls below that experienced by the preceding generation. This change, shown graphically in Figure 7.1, coincides in time with the great reduction in the number of smokers among men and is a justification, in public health terms, of the activities of the anti-smoking lobby.

Table 7.1 Australian male death rates from lung cancer (per 10⁵) for each of three cohorts (average rates per year within the calendar periods specified).

	1950–54	1955–59	1960–64	1965–69	1970–74	1975–79	1980–84	1985–89	1990–93
30–34									
35–39	2								
40–44		9							
45–49	18		24						
50–54		46		58					
55–59	62		101		119				
60–64		130		196		215			
65–69			219		310		322		
70–74				331		425		400	
75–79					440		522		447
80–84						463		522	
85 +							435		455

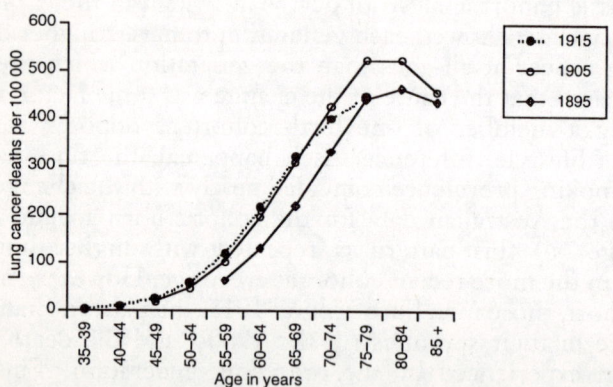

Figure 7.1 *Changes in lung cancer mortality in three cohorts of Australian men, the median year of birth of the cohorts being 1895, 1905 and 1915.*

Infectious Diseases

A cohort analysis may also be applied to morbidity data, such as that relating to infectious diseases. Oliver Lancaster, from the University of Sydney, used the notion of cohorts to explore the relationship between rubella and subsequent deafness.[2] Table 7.2 shows the number of male deaf mutes in New South Wales as enumerated in successive censuses.

In each census the modal age group (the mode is the most frequently occurring value in a set of observations) has been indicated and it is apparent that those who were 10–14 in 1911 form a cohort, and they can be seen again in 1921 (aged 20–24) and in 1933 (aged 30–34). There was a rubella epidemic at the turn of the century and the exposed cohort (babies born at the time) bears the consequences.

Table 7.2 Male deaf mutes in successive NSW censuses.

	Census year		
	1911	*1921*	*1933*
0–4	8	7	7
5–9	34	39	57
10–14	**54**	43	56
15–19	35	30	68
20–24	36	**69**	49
25–29	34	36	44
30–34	24	35	**78**
35–39	35	35	44

Cohort analysis is not confined to disease rates but may also be applied to other characteristics of people that may be thought to be strongly influenced by 'generational differences'. In 'Healthwatch', a study carried out in the Australian petroleum industry, 11 600 employees were interviewed about their lifetime smoking habits.[3] From this information, the prevalences of smoking at different ages, at different times and in different cohorts, could be calculated and results graphed as in Figure 7.2. Were any confirmation of the smoking and lung cancer link required, the demonstration that successive cohorts of men not only have higher lung cancer rates but have higher rates of tobacco smoking would be strong evidence indeed.

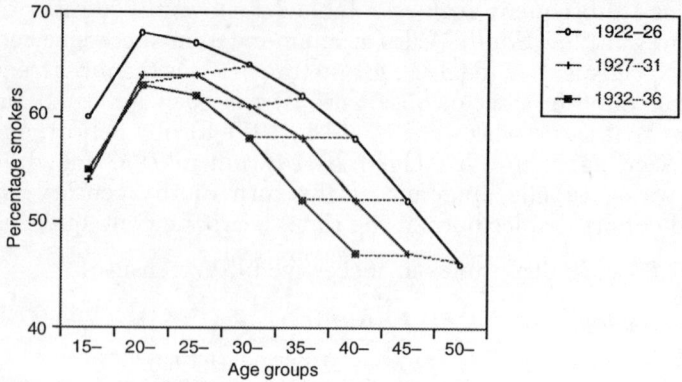

Figure 7.2 *Smoking prevalences at different ages in three generations of Australian men. The key shows the years in which the cohorts were born. Each cohort has generally had a lower prevalence of smoking than the preceding cohort. The dotted lines join points at the same calendar time.*

In each of the examples above a change in an outcome over time was due to lifetime differences between birth cohorts in terms of the occurrence of the risk factor. Sometimes changes are due to some alteration in the environment at a particular calendar time, such as the introduction of a new treatment, and in this case cohort analysis is not appropriate.

In the interpretation of cross-sectional surveys it is sometimes useful to be aware of the possibility of generational differences between cohorts. In 1975 a survey in a Victorian township[4] asked subjects: 'Do you experience headache requiring the regular taking of analgesics (e.g. aspirin)?' Figure 7.3 shows the distribution of positive responses in women by age. There are two possible explanations of the marked age differences: either that the prevalence of headache declines with age, or that different generations perceive a headache differently. It is possible that older women, having grown up in particular social conditions, have lower expectations of being symptom free and regard a headache not so much as a symptom as part and parcel of life. From purely cross-sectional data, age effects cannot be distinguished from cohort effects.

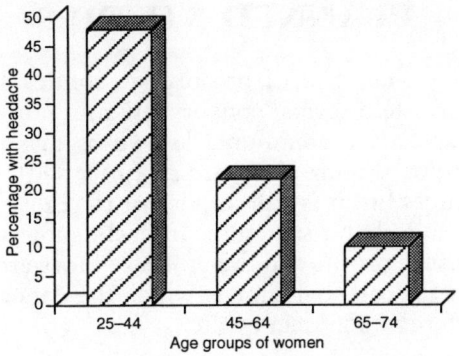

Figure 7.3 *Prevalence of headache for which analgesic is taken, in women by age group.*

'One-off' exposure cohort

An exposure cohort is a body of people who have experienced a common exposure to some chemical or other noxious hazard. The largest exposure cohort ever studied consisted of the inhabitants of Hiroshima and Nagasaki following the atomic bombs in 1945.[5] This long-term observation of the effects of radiation has given many insights into the effects of radiation on health and, in particular, dose-response relationships. An exposure cohort like this, where the exposure was a unique event, may be represented diagrammatically as in Figure 7.4. The initial exposure occurs at time T1 when all the population are exposed, and we assume that the average age of the population is 50 years. As time passes members of the cohort die and are not replaced (no more exposure) and the average age of the cohort increases until ultimately all members have died by T2.

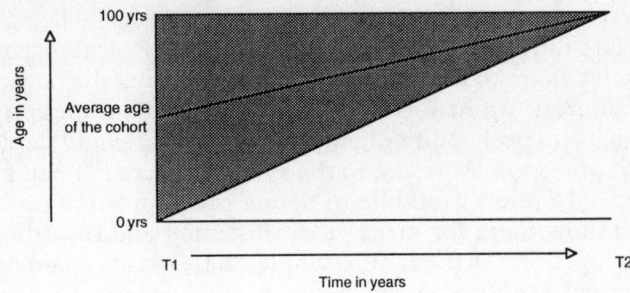

Figure 7.4 *Diagrammatic representation of a 'one off' exposure cohort from time of original exposure (T1) until death of the last member (T2).*

PLANNED STUDIES

Within the general concept of prospective studies are two types of design which Lilienfeld terms 'concurrent' and 'non-concurrent'[6] but which are perhaps more commonly known as historical cohort and prospective cohort. Figure 7.5 (from Lilienfeld) illustrates their apparent differences but it is still important to realise that the designs share the same underlying structure. In each, subjects are defined in terms of an exposure profile and then followed forward over time. The difference lies in the calendar time at which the data are collected and the very real differences in data quality.

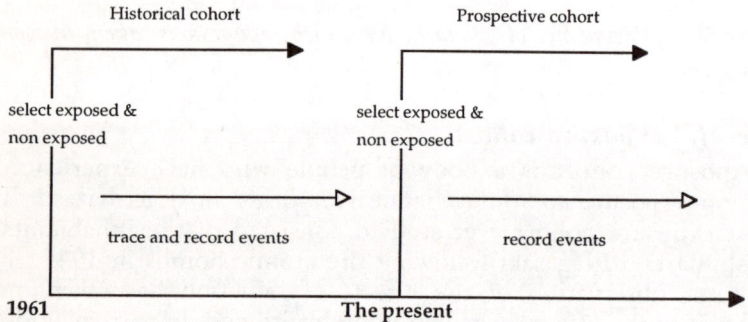

Figure 7.5 *Diagrammatic representation of concurrent and non-concurrent prospective studies.*[6]

If it were decided to investigate some problem now by means of a cohort study, the researcher would have two options. The first of these would be to seek a population defined, say in 1961, as a company payroll, a battalion muster roll, or perhaps the list of new graduates in a professional discipline. The individuals concerned would then need to be characterised in terms of their exposure to what is being studied, and their fate during the years from 1961 to the present discovered by tracing each person to the present day and recording the occurrence of events of interest. An historical cohort study would have been carried out in which the probability of an event occurring could be described in terms of preceding exposure to the agent suspected of being a cause.

The second option would be to define the population as 'here and now' and follow them for many years observing and recording events as they occur. As in the previous example, these events could be related to the original exposure status. A prospective cohort study would be carried out.

Of the designs available for observational epidemiological studies, those with a prospective element provide the strongest evidence of the existence of a cause–effect relationship. Historical cohorts suffer from the fact that the investigator is bound by the limitations of data not only collected many years previously, but also usually collected for quite a different purpose. Nevertheless, the historical cohort study comes at a reasonable dollar cost and the answers to the research question can be available within a matter of months. The prospective cohort study, in contrast, is extremely expensive and the answers are delayed for many years until enough outcome events of interest to permit analysis have accumulated.

A prospective cohort study

'Healthwatch', the prospective study being carried out in the Australian petroleum industry, has been in operation since 1981. The population at risk was defined from payrolls but no direct measures of exposure were available. As is all too common in industrial epidemiology, an accurate job description was used as an indirect measure of exposure. In this study an interview was carried out with each individual to obtain information on such potential confounders as smoking history and previous employment. Outcome events were death by cause and the occurrence of cancer, as reported to the Cancer Registers.

Definitive analyses were delayed until 1991;[7] an interesting interim result was available at the end of 1985. By this time 30 300 person years at risk had accumulated and 94 deaths had occurred. When, as in the top line of Table 7.3, the SMR was calculated using the Australian population as reference, the result was substantially lower than that expected from the rates applying in the general population.

Table 7.3 Deaths of employees of the Australian petroleum industry, age standardised against the Australian population and against Australian Government employees.

Standard	Deaths observed	Deaths expected	SMR (95% CI)
Australian population	94	147	0.64 (0.51–0.78)
Government employees	90*	84	1.07 (0.86–1.31)

* Australian Government data only available for age 65 or less, hence four fewer deaths.

It was believed that this result was due not to the better general health of petroleum industry employees but rather to the operation of the healthy worker effect. This is a selection bias which operates when those people currently in work are compared with the general population, the latter containing those who are unemployable for reasons of ill health. That this explanation is correct is demonstrated in the second line of the table where the SMR has been re-calculated using data relating to Australian government employees as the standard. The difference is substantial and indicates the care that needs to be taken in the choice of a comparison group. In most epidemiological studies, failure to choose an appropriate comparison leads to the incorporation of a wide variety of potential biases into the study design.

Another prospective study was the Honolulu Heart Study[8] in which 7 705 Japanese men without diagnosed coronary heart disease (CHD) were entered into a prospective study between 1965 and 1968. At study entry, information was collected on, among other things, each subject's alcohol intake. After six years of follow-up, the incidence rates for new occurrence of CHD were able to be calculated in terms of that reported alcohol intake. Here the 'exposure' was defined as alcohol consumption and the disease was the occurrence of CHD. Incidence rates are shown in Table 7.4; relative risk has been calculated in respect to the zero consumption group.

Table 7.4 Relative risks of CHD occurrence in terms of reported alcohol consumption in the Honolulu Heart Study.[8]

Alcohol intake (mL per day)	No.	6 yr CHD incidence per 1 000	Relative risk
0	3 565	46.0	1.00
1–6	1 034	41.2	0.90
7–15	962	30.7	0.67
16–39	1 024	26.7	0.58
40 +	1 006	21.2	0.46

Concurrent prospective studies of this nature provide the most powerful and convincing argument for the existence of a true causal relationship. The results from the above study strongly suggest that moderate alcohol consumption has a protective effect as far as CHD is concerned. In a concurrent design one has no doubt about the time relationships, no recall is involved, the outcome events can be specified very precisely, and data on confounding variables can be collected. The problems lie in the inordinate expense of such studies, the length of time that must elapse before answers become available, and in the fact that the nature of the exposure during the follow-up may have changed from that measured at baseline. By the time the study has concluded the original questions may have been forgotten or have become of historical interest only.

An historical cohort study

A much quicker and cheaper way to carry out a prospective study is to define the population as at some time in the past. A question often arises as to whether professional men and women are at greater risk of suicide than others due to the presumed greater stress with which such occupations are associated. A cohort study was carried out in Victoria to examine this question where doctors were the profession concerned.[9]

Between 1950 and 1959, 1279 men and 174 women graduated in medicine from the University of Melbourne and, at the end of 1986, 95.4% of these could be positively identified as being alive or dead. Such completeness of identification is as essential as a good response rate in a cross-sectional survey, for the same reason of excluding selection bias. In a professional group like doctors the follow-up process is immeasurably aided by the existence of State registration boards, which are updated annually and list doctors who are currently paying a registration fee. Table 7.5 shows the SMR (calculated on Victorian population rates of the appropriate calendar years) for suicide of male and female doctors. Also shown are the SMR for all mental disorders including drug and alcohol dependence, and in addition the all cause SMR.

The very low SMR for all causes in both male and female doctors represents an extreme of the healthy worker selection effect, an effect which in this particular example includes the self-selection of members of the higher socio-economic groups into Australian medical courses. For suicide in men, the death rate is greater than would be expected from the general population rates applying, but the confidence limits are wide as would be expected from the small number of these deaths. This confirms that the suicide rate of male doctors is certainly unlikely to be lower than the general population and may possibly be higher. In spite of the low numbers and wide confidence intervals, the data concerning women doctors is most disturbing and suggests an urgent need for further research.

Table 7.5 SMRs and 95% confidence intervals for selected causes of death in male and female Victorian doctors.

Cause of death		Observed deaths	Expected deaths	SMR	95% CI
Male:	All causes	115	194.3	0.59	0.49–0.71
	Suicide	10	8.9	1.13	0.54–2.07
Mental disorders*		3	2.3	1.32	0.27–0.38
Female:	All causes	11	13.0	0.84	0.42–1.51
	Suicide	3	0.6	5.01	1.03–14.7
Mental disorders*		0	0.2		

* Includes drug and alcohol dependence.

Standard practice in the construction of an historical cohort is as shown in Figure 7.6 where each horizontal line represents the time spent by an individual subject as a member of the study. In the 'Healthwatch' project an employee became a member of the cohort either by being in the workforce at the time the study began or by joining that workforce at any time subsequently. In the terms of the figure, subjects **a–e** inclusive were the cohort members, entering at various times, until the analysis point in 1992. A problem with this design lies with the people 'in at the beginning' because they are the survivors; if there is any effect from noxious agents in the work environment then the people in place at the beginning are those who are resistant to that noxious agent or have had as yet little exposure. Other problems relate to the fact that the exposure experienced by the cohort, particularly in the early years of the study, is weighted towards people exposed in earlier periods when conditions may have been very different and were certainly less well documented. A solution lies in the construction of an inception cohort where the criterion for membership is joining the study population *after* the start date. In terms of Figure 7.6 this means that subjects **a** and **d** will be excluded. Although this device avoids the difficulties described above, it does have the disadvantages of smaller PYR in the denominator and younger cohort members less likely to get an age-linked condition (like cancer). Also, since the latent period of a cancer is usually at least 10 years, the number of PYR contributed by subjects with more than 10 years in the exposed category will be correspondingly small. Usually, as with the New South Wales Coalworkers Cancer Surveillance Program,[10] the decision is made on the quality of the available data from which the cohort is to be constructed. In the latter study it proved impossible to be certain that individuals were actually in the workforce on 1 January 1973 so the decision was made to restrict membership to those people who joined the industry on or after that date.

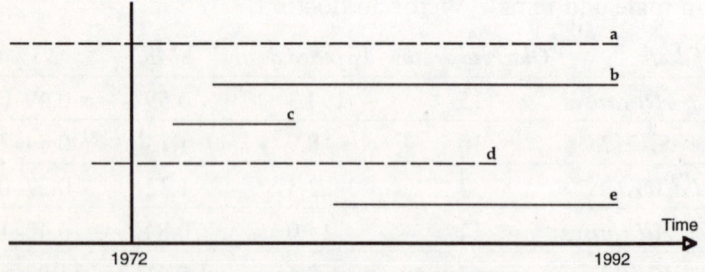

Figure 7.6 *Historical cohorts and inception cohorts.*
Note: Each horizontal line represents a single subject.

EXERCISES

Exercise 7.1

Synthetic mineral fibres (SMFs) are a most valuable material because they have been introduced as 'safe' substitutes for asbestos. SMFs as 'wool' are derived from rock, rock and slag, and glass. Glass filament which is produced as a continuous filament is also classified as an SMF. The worldwide annual production of these materials is some 14 million tonnes. Recently this widely used material has come under suspicion, and indeed has been publicised in Australia and elsewhere, as the 'new asbestos'. As a consequence, an international historical cohort study was carried out to determine whether occupationally determined exposure to SMF was associated with an increased risk of developing cancer of the lung. There were not only many countries involved but also often more than one production site in each country. Table 7.6 shows the countries involved, the years in which the manufacture of SMF began, the type of SMF and the final year of mortality follow-up.

1. In this study how would you define the start date of the cohort?
2. At the end of the period of observation, what will be the denominator and how will this be calculated?
3. In this study it was proposed to pool all the results. Give two reasons why you might be reluctant to do this.

Table 7.6 Contributors to a multinational cohort study of synthetic mineral fibres and lung cancer.[11]

Year of starting production	Country	Type of process	End of follow-up
1937	Denmark	Rock & slag	1982
1941	Finland	Glass wool	1981
1940	Norway	Rock & slag wool	1982
1948	Norway	Rock & slag wool	1982
1950	Norway	Rock wool	1982
1933	Sweden	Rock & slag wool	1982
1935	Sweden	Glass wool	1982
1938	Sweden	Rock & slag wool	1982
1943	United Kingdom	Glass wool	1983
1946	United Kingdom	Glass filament	1982
1941	Germany	Rock wool	1983
1946	Italy	Glass wool	1983
1961	Italy	Glass filament	1983

Exercise 7.2

In the cohort study being carried out in the petroleum industry, preliminary analysis of the occurrence of cancer of the lymphopoietic and haematopoietic tissues showed a relationship to the time of first employment in the industry. This is shown graphically in Figure 7.7 where the age-adjusted relative risks of this cancer are shown for different times of first employment, with the rate of occurrence of cancer where the first employment was between 1975 and 1984 being set at unity. Note that the number of these cancers is small and the relative risks correspondingly imprecise.

An obvious interpretation of Figure 7.7 is that, in this industry, occupationally determined exposure to chemical agents capable of inducing such cancer has been greatly reduced over the last 40 years. This is undoubtedly true but can you think of another possible interpretation which would be less comforting?

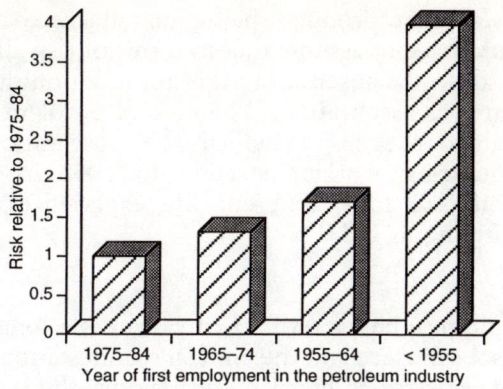

Figure 7.7 *Relative risk of lympho-haematopoietic cancer in petroleum industry employees by length of service in the industry.*

Exercise 7.3

The Natural Feeding Association (NFA) is a voluntary organisation located in a faraway country, whose purpose is to encourage breastfeeding. In that country the NFA has been in existence since 1920 and currently enrols some 4 000 women each year, each of whom has been recently pregnant and who was breastfeeding her child at the time of enrolment. Since 1970 the membership lists have been computerised and include name, address at time of enrolment, age, number of children, and husband's occupation. The country in question has maintained a population-based cancer registry since 1978 which is accessible to bona fide researchers. The country's death registers are well maintained and accessible.

Could an historical cohort study be set up using the NFA register, to test the hypothesis 'that breastfeeding protects against subsequent risk of developing breast cancer'?

ANSWERS

Exercise 7.1

1. The start date refers not to countries but to individuals who are being observed. The start date is thus the date that each person enters the industry.
2. The denominator will consist of the sum total of the person years of exposure contributed by each member of the cohort from the time of his entry to industry until either his death, occurrence of lung cancer (in an incidence study), or the calendar time at which observation ceases.

3. There are different products being manufactured and thus any pooling would have to assume that in terms of risk all types of fibre were identical. In the absence of other information this would seem a most hazardous assumption. The second problem relates to the different calendar times at which the observations started in different countries; workers starting in 1941 in Germany are certainly going to have different life experiences compared to Swedes beginning in 1933!

Exercise 7.2
One of the biological characteristics of cancer is a long latent period between a causal exposure and the clinical manifestation of the cancer. In the case of asbestos induced mesothelioma this latent period is thought to be some 30 years but more usually the median latent period for environmentally induced cancer is about 15 years. If the latent period in the case of this cancer is 15–20 years, then most of the cancers would not have manifested in employees who had started after the 1960s.

Exercise 7.3
It would certainly be quite feasible to set up an historical cohort and produce data on the rate of occurrence of breast cancer in women who had breastfed at least one of their babies. One could also control for a number of potential confounders, such as age at time of feeding, social class and number of children. The problem is 'compared with what?'. It would be necessary to know the rate of occurrence of breast cancer in women who had never breastfed and such data is just not available. It is conceivable that a case-control study could be designed but the problem of controls would not be easily overcome. On the other hand, if the focus of the question was on the relationship (if any) between protection from breast cancer and the amount of breastfeeding, then the NFA data could form a useful cohort.

CHAPTER EIGHT

CASE–CONTROL STUDIES

I n a case–control study the subjects are selected on the basis of their disease status: cases have the disease of interest and controls do not. This is in contrast to the cohort or follow-up study described in the previous chapter, in which subjects are selected in terms of their exposure status, and followed up over time, with respect to the disease outcome.

Cases may come from a population-based register (such as a cancer registry), a survey, or from hospitals or clinics. Controls are chosen from the same population as the cases. To qualify as a potential control, a person needs to be free of the disease of interest and to be someone who would appear as a case in the study if he or she contracts the disease under study. For example, if our cases were people who had been admitted to hospital with stroke, then our controls should be chosen from people who, if they had suffered a stroke, would be admitted to the same hospital. The controls may then be compared to the cases in terms of past exposure to a presumed causal agent, either by survey or by study of records.

There is a sharp difference between cohort and case–control studies in the way subjects are selected, and this has meant historically that the two designs were regarded as being quite different. In reality, the requirement that cases and controls come from the same population at risk means that the case–control study is not as dissimilar from the cohort study as one might think. The layout of a case–control study is as follows:

Table 8.1 Layout of case–control data.

	Cases	Controls
Exposed	a	b
Not exposed	c	d
Total	a+c	b+d

Cases are ideally found by considering all occurrences of the disease of interest which arise in the population at risk over a period. To obtain controls, our aim should be to sample from the same population at risk, in such a way that the sample is representative of the exposure distribution in that population. This is the basic idea, although of course cases arise and controls are chosen over time, and the exposure distribution may change with time, so that in practice the time dimension is important too. For a detailed explanation the reader is referred to Rothman.[1]

From these data we obtain the classic estimate of elevated risk in a case–control study, the odds ratio (OR):

$$OR = \frac{a/b}{c/d} = \frac{ad}{bc}$$

This odds ratio is an estimate of the rate ratio for disease, comparing exposed to unexposed. This works because the numbers of controls, exposed and unexposed, are in proportion to the numbers of exposed and unexposed in the population (or, more precisely, in proportion to the person years in the exposed and unexposed categories).

The term 'odds' comes from gambling—the odds of an event are the probability of the event divided by the probability that it does not occur. Thus, if the odds for a horse winning the Melbourne Cup are 10 to 1 against it is implied that its estimated chance of winning is 1/11 (and losing, 10/11).

In a case–control study, then, the ratio a/c is the sample odds of a case being exposed, since the proportion of cases exposed is $a/(a+c)$ and the proportion not exposed is $c/(a+c)$. Hence the odds ratio is, from one point of view, the ratio of the odds of exposure in the cases to the odds of exposure in the controls. But by far the more useful way to think about the odds ratio in a case–control study is that described above— it is an estimate of the rate ratio, or relative risk, of interest. There are a number of important features of a case–control study.

1. It is critical that the selection of the controls is not influenced by their exposure status. Otherwise, the controls give us a distorted picture of the exposure distribution in the population at risk, and the odds ratio is biased.

2. It is not possible to be sure that a control does not have the disease in a sub- or pre-clinical form, nevertheless it is important that the potential control has not been diagnosed with the disease. Interestingly, this implies that the disease should not have been searched for more aggressively in the cases than in the controls.

3. Controls need to be selected throughout the period of case accrual and not, for example, at the end of it. This is so that the selection of

controls accurately mirrors the person years distribution among exposed and unexposed, which may change over the period of case accrual.

4. Separate estimates of incidence rates in the exposed and unexposed are not possible in a case–control study.

BIAS IN CASE–CONTROL STUDIES

The key assumption in the calculation of odds ratio from a case–control study is that the cases and controls have been selected solely in terms of their having or not having the disease. If there was any possibility of the subjects having been selected in terms of their likelihood of being exposed or not exposed then the risk estimates could be quite wrong and misleading. Whilst it is most unlikely that any investigator would select in this way deliberately, if we get our cases and controls from a hospital or clinic such selection could be operating unbeknown to the investigator.

Consider a hypothetical situation where the occurrence of attacks of asthma in a particular community was thought to have been due to a warehouse fire in the locality which had produced fumes and pollution. A case–control study was done in the local hospital with the cases being people admitted with a diagnosis of asthma and the controls being people of the same age, sex and area of residence, admitted with a diagnosis other than asthma. The exposure of interest was fumes from the fire and the results were as shown in Table 8.2.

Table 8.2 Hospital-derived cases and controls.

	Case (asthma)	Control (no asthma)
Exposed to fumes	5	15
Not exposed	18	219
Total	23	234

The odds ratio (by cross-multiplying) is 4.1, suggesting that people with an attack of asthma were four times as likely to have been exposed to the fumes as were people without asthma. That is to say, one of the elements of Bradford Hill's criteria of causation—a strong association—has been established.

Following this, a prevalence study was carried out of all people living in the locality, using the same definitions of 'asthma' and 'no asthma', and from the data came Table 8.3.

Table 8.3 Community-derived cases and controls.

	Case (asthma)	Control (no asthma)	
Exposed to fumes	17	596	613
Not exposed	184	6 450	6 634
Total	*201*	*7 046*	*7 247*

The calculated odds ratio is 1, that is, no association is present between exposure to fumes and having an attack of asthma. The hospital-based case–control study suggested a causal relationship, but the population-based study failed to confirm it. This paradox probably came about because general practitioners, faced with a patient with asthma, might have been more likely to recommend hospital admission if that patient had been exposed to fumes (greater likelihood of complications perhaps) than if they had not. The result was a distortion of the true exposed/non-exposed ratio in the cases, relative to the controls, which produced a false association of disease with exposure. This is a particular example of selection bias where patients are being selected for hospital admission on criteria other than the severity and nature of the illness.

Other sources of bias are more common, one in particular being that of differential recall between cases and controls. If one were carrying out a study of cervical cancer, then questions on sexual history would be very differently received by the cases and the controls. The cases would regard the question as being relevant and important, but it is unlikely that the controls would give as thoughtful a reply. Another problem arises with population-based cancer case–control studies where only too frequently, by the time the investigator knows about the cancer occurrence, the unfortunate case has died. Information can then only be second-hand as to life experiences (from relatives) and this information is not comparable to the first-hand account given by living controls. In industrial studies the control is at times chosen as a workmate, in which case it is likely that a number of work exposures will be common to both the case and the control. A similar difficulty may arise with 'best friend' controls as the best friend usually shares a similar lifestyle with the case. Situations of this nature where cases and controls are inadvertently matched on the presence or absence of the 'cause', or more usually some factor closely associated with it, are known as overmatching.

TWO CASE–CONTROL STUDIES

....

Case 1

Like all military organisations from historic times to the present, the Royal Australian Air Force (RAAF) requires its recruits to undergo basic military training. Such training is intense and the recruits, even though they are fit young men and women, frequently experience musculoskeletal injury ranging from the trivial to the serious. A case–control study of such injury in recruits, serious enough to delay course completion or to require course postponement, was carried out in a RAAF training facility in South Australia.[2] The cases were the 238 recruits who had suffered such an injury between 1 January 1985 and 31 December 1990 (2.7% of the population at risk). The 629 controls were randomly selected from those recruits who, over the same time period, had not experienced such injury. Cases and controls were thus defined and the 'exposures' of interest were various characteristics of the recruits and their environment as recorded when they entered the RAAF. It is interesting to note here that whilst the original data collection at the entry medical examination could be described as a survey, the passage of time as events occur is a characteristic of a longitudinal study yet, since the cases and controls were defined in terms of the presence or absence of disease, this study is correctly described as being of the case–control variety.

The initial analysis was bivariate with four-fold tables being drawn up as in Table 8.1 (page 79). Exposed and not exposed were defined as possessing or not possessing some characteristic, such as a calendar year of basic training, previous levels of physical activity, gender, or season of the course, and odds ratios were calculated. The relationship of those variables whose odds ratios were at least statistically significant at the 5% level were further examined in a multivariate logistic regression model. The latter concept is more advanced than appropriate for this text and it will suffice to say that an odds ratio from such an analysis is an estimate of the true odds ratio where the effect of all the other variables being examined is 'controlled'. Some of the more important results from this analysis are shown in Table 8.4 as odds ratios with their 95% confidence intervals (CI).

Table 8.4 Odds ratio and 95% CI of a number of possible 'causes' of musculoskeletal injury in RAAF recruits.

	Smoking	Low activity	Medium activity	Winter*	Female	Previous injury
Odds ratio	1.39	1.83	1.58	2.02	2.44	2.65
95% CI	0.98–1.39	0.94–3.43	0.86–2.80	1.41–2.93	1.50–3.92	1.79–3.91

* As opposed to other seasons of recruitment.

One of the more striking findings in this study is illustrated in Figure 8.1 where calendar year is considered as the 'exposure'. Since neither the course itself nor the type of recruit had changed over this time, the investigators considered no less than five possibilities:

1. a change in the culture whereby the reporting of injuries had become more acceptable;
2. improved diagnosis by medical staff whereby injuries were increasingly identified correctly.
3. the course becoming more arduous than in previous times;
4. the recruits somehow becoming more susceptible to injury;
5. a changed perception of musculoskeletal injury and its importance so that injuries were reported that previously would have been ignored.

There is no evidence to support any of the above hypotheses yet over approximately the same time period there was, in the civilian Australian population, an epidemic of what was originally called repetition strain injury (RSI) and later known as occupational overuse syndrome. This was thought by some[3] to be a form of 'social pathogenesis' and it was suggested that some rather tenuous support could be given to the fifth hypothesis above by drawing an analogy with this syndrome.

Hypotheses, and the design of observational studies intended to test them, are limited by the knowledge possessed by the investigator. In the present study the finding that a major influence on the rate of occurrence of injury was the year in which basic training was undertaken evidently came as a surprise and no satisfactory explanation can be offered. Recognising that this finding was possibly the most important outcome of the study, in terms of generating hypotheses for further work, the authors subtitled their paper 'Is there a social element of injury pathogenesis?'.

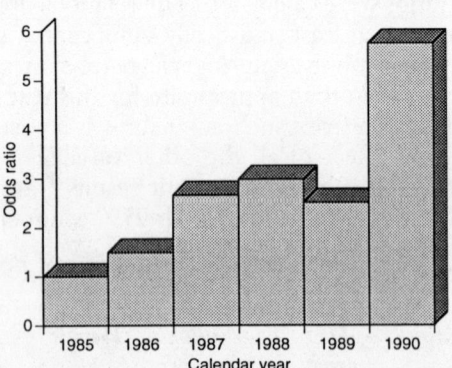

Figure 8.1 *Relationship between calendar time and occurrence of injury in RAAF recruits on basic training courses (odds ratios for calendar years, relative to 1985 as baseline).*

Case 2

You are a physician in a large metropolitan hospital and have an interest in asthma. Over the first six months of the year there were thirteen young asthmatics admitted to your hospital who died within an hour of admission; over the previous six months there had been only two such cases. All but three of the thirteen asthmatics who died were taking the combination of drug A and drug B. From your general knowledge you know that there has been a great increase in the popularity of this combination among the doctors in your area. You are naturally anxious to alert the profession to a possibly dangerous drug combination yet, on the other hand, don't want to falsely incriminate a potentially useful therapy. Bearing in mind that you want an answer fairly quickly, a case–control study would be the design of choice.

Cases are the 13 asthmatics who died after hospital admission. Controls are 26 asthmatics who did not die after admission. Two controls were chosen for each case in such a way as to ensure that cases and controls are balanced for age, sex, severity and week of admission.

In Table 8.5 the previous drug usage of the cases and controls is compared. Of the asthmatics who died 10/13 (77%) were on the suspect drug combination as opposed to 12/26 (46%) of the controls. The odds ratio is 3.9, suggesting that asthmatics on the drug combination are about four times as likely to die as those not on these drugs.

Table 8.5 Drug usage in asthmatic patients who died after hospital admission (cases) and in similar patients who did not die (controls).

	Cases	Controls	
Drug A + B	10	12	22
Other	3	14	17
Total	13	26	39

Note: Odds ratio = 3.9 (95% confidence interval 0.73–26).

With an odds ratio of this size it would be understandable for someone to jump to the conclusion that the drug combination is dangerous and that doctors should be alerted immediately. The problem is, however, that the numbers are quite small and, as a direct consequence, the 95% confidence interval is wide and includes unity. This means that this apparently strong relationship may have arisen by chance alone. In this clinical situation there are only two possibilities, either:
1. the drug combination is dangerous; or
2. the drug combination is not dangerous.

From carrying out this study, the results of which are shown in Table 8.5, we appear to have landed ourselves in a rather difficult situation. We could be very scientific and say (correctly) that it is not possible to blame the drug combination for the deaths because the 95% confidence limits are so wide that the results could have occurred by chance alone. On the other hand, there is the real possibility that the result did not occur by chance and hence a speedy warning to the profession could result in valuable lives being saved. This dilemma is the result of a poor study design with a failure to take into account all considerations, especially those of sample size.

EXERCISES

Exercise 8.1

Cirrhosis of the liver is a progressive replacement of functioning liver tissue by fibrous tissue, with the ultimate consequence of failure of the liver to carry out its essential metabolic tasks. The most common cause by far is long-standing alcohol misuse. Less commonly it can follow viral infections of the liver and, rarely, other causes such as solvent exposure. The clinical course of cirrhosis extends over many years and in the worst cases ends with liver failure and death.

A case–control study was carried out to determine the risk for Australian men of developing alcoholic cirrhosis as a result of prolonged alcohol misuse at differing levels of consumption.[4] The cases and controls were obtained from patients admitted to either of two large Sydney hospitals and each subject was interviewed. As part of the interview a very detailed history of lifetime alcohol consumption was taken.

1. a) What is the exposure being studied?
   b) What is meant by the term 'risk' both generally and specifically in relationship to this study?
2. In an 'ideal world', with limitless finance, would you choose a case–control design to answer the research question as did the present authors, or would you choose a different type of study? Refer here to the results as reported which are presented in Table 8.6.

The cases were 33 men with newly diagnosed alcoholic cirrhosis of the liver. In 20 of these the diagnosis of alcoholic cirrhosis was established by a liver biopsy; in 13 this test was not carried out due to the risk of severe bleeding. The latter had no relevant history, other than that of alcohol excess, and a definite clinical diagnosis of cirrhosis could be made.

Table 8.6 Odds ratios of men with alcoholic cirrhosis and controls.

Average alcohol intake (grams per day)	No. of cases	No. of controls	Odds ratio
≤ 40 grams	3	78	1
41–80 grams	12	6	52
> 80 grams	18	5	94

3. Do you think it likely that a bias was introduced by the inclusion of cases of alcoholic cirrhosis where that diagnosis was made other than by biopsy?

For each case, three male patients in the same hospital at the same time and of the same age as the identified cirrhotic patient, but with another diagnosis, were chosen for interview as controls.

4. Can you think of any potential bias that the use of hospital inpatients as controls could introduce into the study? What would be the effect of such bias if present?

5.a) Is it possible to calculate the 'attributable risk' of alcohol consumption from the data collected in the present study?

b) Of what type of risk is the odds ratio an unbiased estimate?

c) In Table 8.6 the odds ratio for men whose average intake was between 41 and 80 grams a day is 52. What does this mean? Show by means of a table or in words how the authors calculated this odds ratio.

d) Calculate the odds ratio of the risk of alcoholic cirrhosis in men who drink more than 80 grams of alcohol per day compared to men who drink less than this amount.

With regard to alcoholic liver disease there are two related questions, the answers to which are important to those setting up preventive programs:

> Is it possible to show a reduction in the incidence of alcohol-related liver disease by lowering rather than by prohibiting the use of alcohol?
>
> Is there a threshold value of alcohol intake below which there appears to be no risk of developing alcoholic-related cirrhosis?

6. Do you think that the results of this study would be able to provide an answer to either or both these questions? If not, what kind of study would be required?

ANSWERS

1. a) The exposure being studied is alcohol consumption and since alcoholic cirrhosis relates to long-term consumption, some index of lifetime or other measure of usual drinking will be needed from a dietary history.

   b) Risk is the probability of a hazard (in this case alcohol consumption) being realised as disease manifestation (liver cirrhosis). In this context 'risk' means the probability that a person with a specified alcohol intake will develop alcoholic cirrhosis of the liver.

2. In an ideal world, one would prefer not to choose a case–control design because it would be better to be able to characterise subjects in terms of exposure, that is drinking, than upon outcome, that is cirrhosis. The principal reason is that it would be helpful to know the risk of drinking from all amounts, not just above 40 grams per day. Unfortunately we live in a world where the ideal, that is a longitudinal or prospective study, is only too often unattainable.

3. Probably not. Nevertheless, whilst the included cases certainly had chronic liver failure the 'alcohol' diagnosis in those not biopsied was one of exclusion on the basis of a number of tests. There are causes of liver failure other than alcohol which could have been included in the case set. On balance the risk that the results could have been biased in this way may be regarded as negligible.

4. The usual problem with hospital controls is that, by definition, they must have some disease or other condition. Since alcohol affects so many systems a hospital patient is more likely to be an alcohol abuser than a control derived from say the electoral roll of a community. The risk of bias is not likely to be serious but if present would bias the results in the direction of minimising the risks of alcohol.

5.a) It is not possible to calculate an attributable risk because there is no information about any identifiable population at risk and thus neither the cirrhosis incidence in drinkers or non-drinkers can be measured.

b) Relative risk.

c) That men whose average daily alcohol intake lies between 41 and 80 grams per day have 52 times the risk of having liver cirrhosis than men with an intake of less than or equal to 40 grams per day.

Table 8.7 Four-fold table from which the odds ratio of men drinking > 40 grams of alcohol per day may be calculated.

Alcohol intake	Cases	Controls
Exposed (41–80 grams)	12	6
Not exposed (< 41 grams)	3	78
Total	15	84

OR = 12 × 78 / 6 × 3 = 52

d) Calculation of odds ratio of having liver cirrhosis in men who drink 80 or more grams of alcohol per day compared with men who drink less than or equal to 80 grams per day.

Table 8.8 Four-fold table from which the odds ratio of men drinking > 80 grams of alcohol per day may be calculated.

Alcohol intake	Cases	Controls
Exposed (80 grams +)	18	5
Not exposed (< 80 grams)	15	84
Total	33	89

OR = 18 × 84 / 5 × 15 = 20

6. The design could not answer either question. With regard to the first, the study could only show that a lower intake is associated with a lower risk of cirrhosis. This is not the same as showing that reducing intake on an individual or population basis would be associated with a reduction in cirrhosis occurrence. To demonstrate such an effect would require a randomised trial at the individual level or observation of a mass effect on a population level (which could follow, for example, a great increase in the price of alcohol). The second question could only be answered by a longitudinal study because it really implies collecting the data from which a dose-effect relationship could be studied. For such a task, one would need the risk at levels below 40 grams a day, including zero.

CHAPTER NINE

RANDOMISED CONTROLLED TRIALS

❧

In a randomised controlled trial, subjects in a population are randomly assigned into groups, which receive or do not receive an experimental intervention. The outcomes in the groups are compared. Random allocation, which may be achieved by some randomising device such as coin tossing or random number tables, is to ensure that (within chance variation) the study and control groups are balanced on extraneous variables which may influence the outcome, so removing the problems of confounding that bedevil observational studies. A randomised controlled trial is the most scientifically rigorous method available in epidemiology.

Many of the actions we perform in our day-to-day practice are based on 'clinical impressions'. Nevertheless, without the benefit of evidence that such action does more good than harm, we may not be offering the best advice to the person seeking it. For example, it was thought for some years that hormone injections in pregnancy might prevent miscarriage. A randomised controlled trial was set up by the Medical Research Council (MRC) of the United Kingdom and no difference was found in the outcome in those pregnancies where oestrogens were injected compared with placebo injections.[1] The implications of this are more profound than just realising that an unnecessary treatment practice has been performed for many years—a number of cases of vaginal carcinoma have been observed in the female offspring of women treated with oestrogens in pregnancy.[2] In addition, a long-term follow-up of the women in the MRC trial found an excess of breast cancer in the women given hormone injections.[3] Thus, both the women and their children were exposed to real danger by the use of an unproven therapy.

The controlled trial is a method of assessing the value of interventions and the latter range far wider than the giving of drugs in clinical situations. Further, the method is not restricted to random allocation of individuals because, particularly in the health promotion field, it is often better for whole communities to be allocated either to receive the intervention or to act as controls. In a study of the effectiveness of an anti-smoking campaign in workplaces,[4] eight companies were randomly assigned to receive or not receive an educational programme. Follow-up surveys were carried out at one and six months to determine the effectiveness of the programme. Whilst it may not be feasible to subject every intervention to a controlled trial, some examples follow of how information derived from less rigorous examinations might be misleading.

DIFFICULTIES ARISING FROM NON-RANDOMISED STUDIES

....

Observational studies

'Over the span of seven years, 1962–69, the medical field successively witnessed the discovery, the adoption, and finally the abandonment of gastric freezing as a treatment of duodenal ulcer.'[5] Freezing, by irrigation with coolant at a temperature of −10°C of a balloon positioned in the stomach, was reported by way of a series of uncontrolled clinical observations in 1962. This was a safe, painless and simple form of treatment which made sense in physiological terms in that the secretion of acid by the stomach was reduced. It appeared to give pain relief, was enthusiastically endorsed by many American surgeons and became the standard treatment for duodenal ulcer in many small clinics throughout the United States. It was not until 1969, following the negative reports of well designed randomised double blind, controlled trials,[6] that this form of treatment was abandoned. By this time it has been estimated that at least 2500 freezing machines were in use and countless patients had endured a useless treatment.

It is almost certain that what was being seen in the earlier observational studies was the well known 'placebo' effect. This occurs when the observer, who only too often has a vested interest in the success of the treatment, knows the patient is on the new treatment and unwittingly encourages them to report improvement in symptoms. In a 'single blind' trial the subject does not know whether they are taking the active treatment or the placebo. When the trial is described as 'double blind' this means that neither doctor nor patient knows who is receiving the active treatment. An additional precaution is to build into the trial design objective criteria of success. Both these strategies help to protect the investigator from false rejection of the null hypothesis, thus promoting a useless drug or, conversely, falsely accepting it which denies patients a useful therapy.

Use of 'historical controls'

Not infrequently doctors find that the survival among their patients with some particular condition is better than in earlier times when they may have used a different treatment. The easy assumption that the present therapy is better than that used in the past ignores the possibility that other factors influencing survival may have changed with time. In 1987 the drug zidovudine, or AZT, was introduced and widely adopted in Australia for treatment of acquired immune deficiency syndrome (AIDS). In 1990 a study of the survival times of patients diagnosed before 1987 was compared with those of patients first diagnosed after this time and the latter group had experienced a definite improvement.[7] Whilst this was gratifying to all concerned, the cause may not necessarily have been the use of AZT; a case could be made that better all round management and understanding of the condition over recent years has been the major contributing factor. Over recent years a number of controlled trials, designed to compare AZT with placebo in patients with AIDS, have been carried out but the results are far from clear. One such trial was begun in the United States in 1987, studying the effect of AZT in preventing the onset of dementia,[8] but was prematurely terminated because of ethical concerns. Nevertheless, the data that were collected do suggest a benefit from the drug in lessening the impact of one of the more unpleasant aspects of this condition. In patients who are HIV infected, yet do not have an AIDS defining illness, a review of 10 randomised, double blind, placebo controlled trials completed by mid-1994 suggested that, whilst early initiation of AZT treatment delayed disease progression, the benefit did not seem to be maintained in the longer term.[9]

Difficulties in the correct interpretation of observational studies are not confined to the evaluation of drugs. In the 1970s an organisation called the Samaritans was set up in the UK to dissuade people who were depressed from committing suicide. The towns where Samaritan offices were opened were shown to have a reduced suicide rate within a couple of years of their opening. However, a careful researcher then compared the fall in suicide rates in these towns with that reported in towns of similar geographical location and size but where there were no Samaritan offices. The suicide rates had fallen by the same amount in both sets of towns.[10] The Samaritans were 'taking the credit' for a fall in suicide rates—however an alternative and plausible explanation arose in the fact that the towns' gas supplies had been changed from coal gas to natural gas. Putting one's head into a gas oven supplied by natural gas is not fatal and this was a favourite method of suicide in those days.

Analysis of 'intention to treat'

In any drug trial some people will take the tablets as prescribed and others will not; they will forget, they might be put off by side effects or perhaps they just don't believe in taking drugs. In any case, it has been shown often that those who take the tablets prescribed by the doctor are likely to fare better than those who are not compliant—even if the tablets do not work! A study, of the benefits of a lipid-lowering drug, showed that people who took most of their tablets did better than those who didn't. The curious thing was this pattern was also seen among those who were taking or not taking the placebo.[11] Those who take the tablets are different in certain ways from those who refuse, and it is this 'difference' that, as it often appears to be related to the outcome, acts as a confounding variable. In a randomised drug trial, as long as enough subjects have been recruited the treatment and control groups will be reasonably comparable in all such possible confounders at the beginning of the study and it follows that all comparisons of outcome must be between these original groups. Thus, if the research question is rephrased as an evaluation of the decision to 'offer treatment' as compared with 'not offer treatment' then the results will be unbiased. This will not necessarily be so where the fate of only those who actually took the treatment is considered.

Along similar lines was a study of survival after a myocardial infarction in people randomly allocated to receive a beta-blocker drug immediately after admission to the Coronary Care Unit compared with those given a placebo.[12] In the course of this trial people had to be withdrawn from both arms for a variety of reasons, of which the most important was deterioration in their condition. Hence the survival rate was lower in those who had to be withdrawn. Since more people on the beta-blocker had to be withdrawn than on the placebo, a comparison of those completing the study showed an apparent benefit to those taking the active drug. When all the patients were considered there was no difference between the groups assigned to the different treatments.

POINTS TO CONSIDER WHEN REVIEWING CLINICAL TRIALS

......

1. *Has the appropriate trial design been used?* In this text only the simplest form of trial has been described. In textbooks on the subject,[13] more

complicated designs including multi-centre, cross-over, and sequential trials are dealt with in some depth.

2. *Have the appropriate end points been used?* In a trial of the value of iron therapy in iron deficiency anaemia, even though the haemoglobin levels increased there were no changes in symptoms among those treated.[14] Which is the appropriate end point to the trial— haemoglobin levels or how the patient feels?

3. *Is the follow-up period long enough?* In a study of the value of admitting patients to a special stroke unit, rather than just to a general ward after their cerebrovascular accident, those in the stroke unit had made a significantly better recovery after three months than those admitted to a general ward. By the end of one year this difference had disappeared.[15] Was it worth it?

4. *Consider the general applicability of the results.* A study of the value of admitting patients to a Coronary Care Unit after their myocardial infarction (MI) found that no benefit accrued.[16] Closer study of the paper reveals that, of the available patients with a heart attack, only 20% were entered into the trial and for this reason the results can only apply to a subgroup of all the people who suffer a heart attack. When deciding to apply the results of a trial to a particular patient it is vital to know if the trial actually applied to the kind of patient you are seeing. In many trials there are so many exclusion criteria, or the conditions of the trial are so artificial, that it is difficult to apply the results to normal clinical practice.

5. *Was the number of subjects in the study large enough?* Matters of sample size are discussed in Chapter 13; it will suffice here to quote Pocock[13] '… a very substantial number of patients are needed to establish with any confidence that two treatments have comparable efficacy.'

6. *Was it double blind?*

SOME ETHICAL ISSUES

In a randomised clinical trial (RCT) carried out to evaluate a new or improved form of therapy the central ethical issue is a guarantee that no subject, be they in the treatment or the control group, will be harmed by participation in the trial. From this premise a number of sub-issues arise.

The investigator cannot **know** that one form of treatment is better than another, since then the subjects receiving the inferior treatment would be disadvantaged. The researcher may suspect, believe, ratiocinate, or even have a full quiver of animal experiments showing the superiority of the new treatment, but must not know that in humans one of the treatments is better than the other.

The proposed new treatment must be as safe as can reasonably be known and therefore unlikely to bring harm to the patient. What may be regarded as 'reasonable' of course changes with increasing knowledge. Today no one would carry out an RCT of a drug to be administered to pregnant women without major documentation concerning possible ill effects on the foetus. This has not always been the case.

If there exists a standard or usual treatment for the condition being studied, then it is desirable that this recognised treatment not be withheld from any patient. It follows that patients in both the treatment and the control arms should receive the standard 'current best practice' with the new treatment being added on to one group. Where this is undesirable for any reason, then patients receiving the new treatment should be compared with patients receiving the usual care; special precautions are taken to end the trial quickly should the new treatment prove either better or worse than the standard. This can be done with a sequential design.

The use of a placebo or dummy treatment is only justified either when there is no current treatment available or when the effectiveness of such treatment is in serious doubt. The latter doubt must be shared by the general medical community, as opposed to being a belief only held by its proponent.

Consent is an important matter. As a general rule all subjects need to be **fully** informed about all aspects of the trial before being asked to participate. In today's climate, when in doubt as to how much a subject should be told, always err on the side of giving too much information. On fairly rare occasions, to divulge fully to a subject all aspects of the study would render it scientifically unsound. Such experiments might include studies of behavioural conditioning, where the subject would not necessarily be informed of the response expected from a specific stimulus. In such circumstances full documentation should be supplied to the appropriate Institutional Ethics Committee and the problem discussed with the Committee. The protocol would be expected to contain details of how, at the end of the study, the subjects would be informed.

Usually in trials of medical intervention the subject is a patient under the care of a doctor for the condition in question and it is usually unwise for the investigator to be the doctor with the responsibility of care. If by the nature of things this situation cannot be avoided, a third party should be entrusted with the task of seeking consent. Where the doctor caring for the patient is not the investigator, then the responsible doctor needs to be fully informed about the proposed study and to agree that the subject may be approached.

Whilst clinical trials with 'hard' or objective end points are generally preferred because of the elimination of bias, quite often an end point with a large subjective component is necessary. Under these circumstances a double blind trial, where neither researcher nor subject knows who is receiving active treatment, is the preferred design. The ethical problem lies in the fact that, by the very nature of things, the subject is usually suffering from some medical condition which could get worse during the course of the study. It is principally for this reason that the researcher and treating doctor should be different people, independent of each other, because the doctor needs to be able to break the code at any time if the subject's health is at risk. Such an action ends that subject's participation in the study and the analysis of the results will need to take account of this.

EXERCISES

Exercise 9.1

Accidental or intended drug overdose is an important part of the work of general hospitals and constitutes 1% of all admissions to the Princess Alexandra Hospital, Brisbane—from which came the data for the present study. The 'standard' treatment of most drug overdoses (the exceptions are corrosive substances and hydrocarbon products) consists of a combination of stomach emptying followed by administration of activated charcoal. The former procedure means vomiting induced by the drug ipecacuanha in conscious patients or by washing out the stomach by way of a tube passed through the mouth in those with reduced alertness. These alternatives are not only quite unpleasant for the subject but for the last 20 years doubts have been cast on their effectiveness. A study of this was reported in 1995 and the authors' abstract of that study follows.[17] Note that those subjects whose stomach was emptied (by vomiting or by tube) are referred to as belonging to the 'emptied group' (E). In those subjects where vomiting was induced by a drug (ipecacuanha), over half also vomited their first dose of charcoal compared with only a quarter of the 'non-emptied group' (NE).

Abstract[17]

Objective: to test the hypothesis that administration of activated charcoal is as efficacious and safe as the combination regimen of gastric emptying plus charcoal in adults after acute oral overdose.

Design: prospective randomised controlled trial, with subjects presenting on odd numbered dates allocated to the emptied group (E), and those on even numbered dates to the non-emptied group (NE).

Setting: Princess Alexandra Hospital, Brisbane (a tertiary referral hospital), which serves an adult urban community, between 4 January 1988 and 11 June 1990.

Subjects: consecutive patients (13 years or older) who presented to the Emergency Department after ingesting an overdose of one or more compounds able to be adsorbed by activated charcoal.

Interventions: all patients received charcoal by the oral or nasogastric route. Those in the E group also had gastric emptying by ipec-induced emesis or gastric lavage.

Outcome measures: clinical course during the first six hours after treatment began, length of hospital stay, complications.

Results: 876 patients were eligible for the study. There were no significant differences between the E and NE groups in age and sex distribution, severity of the overdose or other characteristics, except the mean interval between presentation and administration of charcoal (91 min [standard deviation, 52] for E group and 55 min [standard deviation, 41] for the NE group; P = 0.0001). There were no significant differences in outcome when the groups were stratified for severity of the overdose or into subgroups that presented sooner or later than one hour after ingestion.

Conclusions: gastric emptying can be omitted from the treatment protocol for adults after acute oral overdose.

From the information given in the abstract above, together with your general knowledge of the problem, consider the following questions.
1. Is the topic one of importance to the individual, the hospital, the community?
2. Is the design chosen, that is the RCT, an appropriate one to answer the research question and why? Does the very nature of the problem imply constraints on an ideal RCT design and, if so, give an example of one such constraint.
3. 'Ethical approval was given by the Princess Alexandra Hospital Ethics Committee.'[17] What problems do you think that committee might have had to wrestle with? Considering the section in this chapter on the ethics of the RCT, what do you think that your view would have been had you been a member of the committee?
4. The crux of an RCT lies in the fact that subjects (or groups) are randomly allocated to the appropriate comparison groups. Do you agree that subject allocation was indeed by a truly random process giving confidence that, apart from the operation of chance, any comparisons made between the two groups would be unbiased?

If you do not agree explain your reasons and state whether these doubts would cause you to reject the authors' conclusions.

5. The reason for random allocation is to eliminate the possibility of any systematic difference between the groups in terms of possible confounding variables. In the abstract it is noted that the mean time between arrival at hospital (presentation) and charcoal administration was 91 minutes in the E group and 55 minutes in the NE group. Assuming that charcoal is an effective treatment, does this time difference constitute a confounding variable and, if so, how could such confounding happen in a properly randomised study? In any case what should be done about it?

6. The report of this study was accompanied by an editorial in the *Medical Journal of Australia*[18] where the following comment was made. 'The study is sufficiently large to conclude that routine gastric emptying as initial treatment of drug overdose is not required. In most cases, the administration of activated charcoal and supportive care are sufficient treatment.' Which parts of this statement are supported by the data gathered in the study and which are not? Although agreeing generally with the study's conclusions, the reviewers were not entirely happy with one further aspect of the study design. What do you think that this might have been, and with whom would you agree?

Exercise 9.2

A study of different types of cushion in relation to pressure sores in the elderly was carried out.[19] The authors' abstract follows.

Abstract[19]

In a modified sequential trial, we randomly assigned 288 elderly patients who were assessed to be of high risk of developing pressure sores (Norton score < 14) to use slab foam or customised contoured foam cushions in their wheelchairs for three months. A total of 359 sores developed in 169 (68%) of the 248 at risk patients who completed the study. The sores were mostly of the persistent erythema level (57%) in severity and took an average of 28 days to heal. No significant differences were found in overall incidence, severity, or healing time of the sores of the patients who used the slab (n=85) or the contoured (n=84) cushions. Significantly more sores developed in the area of ischial tuberosities in the slab cushion group and in the sacrococcygeal region of the contoured cushion group. Age and severe malnourishment were found to be associated with the incidence of sores but the number of hours seated daily and other patient characteristics were not related. We concluded that customised cushions should be offered only to those elderly patients who do not have a tendency to slide in the chair.

1. What is the hypothesis being tested in this study?
2. What is the type of study being used here and what are its advantages over other study designs?
3. What does the word 'sequential' mean in this context and under what circumstances is a sequential design generally preferred?
4. In the first paragraph of this paper, the authors criticise the work of other authors in that their studies 'lack control of the placebo effect'. What is meant by this expression and how might it operate in a study of the present nature? Do you think that such a placebo effect is likely to be present, given the information you have had so far?
5. The subjects were residing in a 430 bed 'extended care facility' in Vancouver, Canada between 1989 and 1990. They needed to be over 60 years of age, free of any skin breakdown for at least two weeks before the study, considered to be at high risk of a pressure sore, and sitting for at least four consecutive hours a day in a wheelchair. How confident are you of the external validity of this study, that is to what degree do you think that its results could be generalised to your own geographic area and to the sort of old person in that region who is likely to be in need of protective cushions?
6. In Table 9.1 certain characteristics of the subjects are considered. The presence of each of these is likely to influence the occurrence of pressure sores but do you think that in the study they are likely to be confounding variables? Explain.

Table 9.1 Some characteristics of the subjects in the trial groups.

	Slab group	*Contour group*	*Total*
Malnourished	5	5	10
Incontinent	35	31	66
Oedema	19	19	38

7. During the trial 40 subjects 'dropped out' (22 died) and these were evenly distributed between the two groups. How do you think the analysis should be done so that the information contributed by these dropouts is not lost?
8. At the end of the study the results on the 248 remaining subjects were actually presented in two ways:
   a) incidence of pressure sores: 184/125 in the slab group and 175/123 in the contoured group;
   b) proportion of subjects developing any sores: 85/125 in the slab group and 84/123 in the contour group.
   Which of these two ways of presenting the results do you think is most appropriate and why?

9. From the above result it is apparent that there was no meaningful difference in the occurrence of pressure sores between the two groups. Nevertheless it was noted that of the subjects who did develop a pressure sore, those using the contoured cushion were more likely to develop the sore in the sacrococcygeal region while those using the slab were more likely to develop the sore over the ischial tuberosities. The authors' conclusion was as follows: '...Thus, considering the expense that is involved, the contoured cushions should be offered to very select elderly patients. The selected patients would be those who are at risk of pressure sores in the area of the ischial tuberosities only...'. Comment.

ANSWERS

Exercise 9.1

1. The efficacy, and relative unpleasantness, of any form of treatment that we as individuals are to be subjected to is extremely important to us as consumers. From a health service point of view any condition that accounts for 1% of hospital admissions, tying up staff and scarce resources, is important to that hospital. Most people would agree that because of the ubiquity of drugs and the frequency of overdoses in our society the topic is important. Nevertheless, these latter comments come from general knowledge and not from information provided in the abstract nor in the body of the report. The importance of some conditions to the community can only be answered from population-based data, rather than from data collected from any single hospital serving that population.
2. The research question concerns a form of treatment and any alternative to a randomised trial would carry all the difficulties in interpretation described earlier. It is as appropriate to use the RCT technique to evaluate a physical treatment as it is for drug therapy. One constraint on the design is the impossibility of single or double blinding. This is true for all treatments that involve 'hands on', including surgical interventions. While this by no means excludes such treatments from trials it does put the onus on the investigators to use objective outcomes that cannot be influenced by knowledge on the part of doctor or client as to the type of treatment the latter may be receiving.
3. The core ethical problem lies with the matter of informed consent. Almost all subjects will have impaired reasoning powers by virtue of the drug they have taken and this may range from 'vagueness' to deep coma. Many of the subjects will have made a deliberate decision to end their lives and thus asking for their consent to implement one or the other life-saving procedure certainly raises difficulties—suppose

they refused either? In a number of suicide attempts the subject would be regarded by some as being of unsound mind, possibly temporarily, and hence the validity of their consent could be open to doubt. Any decision you might have made, had you been on the committee in question, would depend to a large extent on the way you balance gain to the community against loss of individual autonomy. With regard to possible disadvantage to control patients it is clear that every patient received good care and the absence of the stomach-emptying procedure in some would not appear to be important in the view of either the investigators or the authorities quoted. Difficult discussions of this nature would have been regarded as totally unnecessary by most investigators 20 to 30 years ago.

4. The question is whether a doctor could in some way control or influence a patient's admission so that it occurred on an even numbered date as opposed to an odd numbered date. Certainly people do not arrange the timing of their overdoses to suit clinical investigators, and further it would be reprehensible for a doctor to delay an urgent admission on these grounds. Nevertheless, for patients arriving in the Emergency Department at, say 11.55 pm, the recorded date of their admission could be influenced by staff members' belief as to which treatment was the best—that given on odd dates or that given on even dates. A reasonable person would accept that the randomisation technique was adequate.

5. Assuming that charcoal is effective, the fact that the E group received their charcoal on average 36 minutes later than the NE group would at first glance fulfil the criteria for a confounding variable. To be certain that all potential confounding variables are going to be evenly balanced on both sides of a trial requires a very large number of subjects and when the number is small or, as in the case of the present study, moderate, then 'chance confounding' is always a possibility. Where the effect of a known possible confounder would be large then randomisation within strata, defined on the presence or absence of that variable, provides protection against a distorted result from such confounding that might occur by chance.

The circumstances of the present study are different in that it is likely that part of the delay may have been linked to one of stomach emptying treatments rather than being an unexpected chance finding. This is suggested in the paper where it is noted that 55% of the NE group vomited their first dose of charcoal as compared to only 13% in the E group. This would delay the administration of an effective dose of charcoal. The investigators handled this difficulty by basing their interpretation on a comparison between two treatments, one being charcoal and the other being a 'package' of charcoal plus stomach emptying with delayed charcoal administration being an inseparable part of that package.

6. The research question was designed to test the proposition that gastric emptying provides no additional advantage to patients who are being treated with charcoal which would allow the efficacy of charcoal to be tested against 'no charcoal'. The study does not address the question of the value of charcoal plus supportive treatment against supportive treatment alone.

In the editorial, comment was made that the relative toxicity of various drugs and drug groups in overdose is quite variable, so that 'not all antihistamines or all tricyclic antidepressants are equally toxic in overdose'.[18] As a consequence, studies on drug overdose should take into account the specific drug in question rather than lumping all drugs into a single category. An argument against this might be that when a doctor makes decisions concerning first line emergency measures, the exact drug taken may not be known. As a consequence the most useful research question might be the one posed by the investigators in this study.

Exercise 9.2

1. That in elderly patients at high risk of developing pressure sores there is no difference between use of foam cushions that have been contoured to fit the individual and cushions that are simple slabs of foam.

2. A randomised controlled clinical trial. The major advantages are that there is a contemporary control group and that all possible confounding factors, both known and unknown, are equally balanced between the two groups.

3. Generally patients enter a trial one by one and are allocated randomly to receive the treatment or to be a control. As a consequence, the earlier a patient is enrolled in the trial the earlier will results on that patient be available to the investigators. Should a treatment prove to be very successful in comparison with a standard treatment then one would wish to stop the trial and change all the control subjects to the new treatment. Conversely, where the new treatment was obviously worse one would wish to change all those receiving it back to the standard therapy. This means that interim analyses must be performed before the trial is scheduled to end, and decisions made that can be both clinically and statistically justified. This is more complex than it appears and the reader is referred to a textbook such as Pocock[13] for a full discussion of the problem. Sequential trials are preferred when, for any reason, it is important to know as early as possible about superiority or inferiority of the therapy under examination. The cost is a higher risk of making wrong decisions because of insufficient data, and this needs to be weighed against the need for early decisions.

4. An effect due not to the intrinsic benefits of a treatment but rather due to other things like the attention being paid to a person, a good feeling due to being treated with something special, and so forth. In the present case patients might feel that a contoured cushion, being more expensive than a slab and more 'personalised', would be more effective and this belief would colour their responses. In the present study a placebo effect is not likely because of the objective nature of the end point.

5. Very confident in principle because in the patient selection there was no obvious bias and, furthermore, the occurrence or not of a pressure sore is essentially a mechanical event. This should not vary much between countries, or communities within a country. Nevertheless, the patient characterisation is quite specific and one would be unable to generalise outside this age range and 'kind of patient'.

6. Table 9.1 shows that for three important possible confounding variables there is no meaningful difference between the two groups being studied. Thus, although these factors may be causal, in the present study they are not confounders. This is a direct result of the randomisation.

7. The subjects who dropped out were being observed from randomisation to the time they dropped out. During this time they were at risk of developing pressure sores and, had such a sore been noted, it should have counted as an end point. The time between randomisation and dropout would be reckoned in person months and added to the denominator.

8. The proper comparison is between the proportion of subjects who developed sores, not the number of sores in the groups. The problem is that 'sores' are not independent; the occurrence of a sore is very dependent on personal characteristics and, therefore, the probability of a person who already has a sore getting a second one is far greater than the probability of a person with no sores getting their first.

9. In this study no difference was found between the type of cushion and the likelihood of a pressure sore occurring. Thus, even if we could identify those 'at risk of pressure sores in the area of the ischial tuberosities only...' the data from the trial indicates that they would get their sore somewhere else. The situation is analogous to a drug trial, where death was the measure of failure, and the result that the 'all cause mortality' was the same in the two groups. Should examination of the data show that the patients given the drug had fewer heart attacks than those given a placebo, then it follows that they must have died of something else. A drug whose only benefit is to alter what is written on one's death certificate is unlikely to have wide appeal—it is a bit like shifting your deck chair on the *Titanic*.

CHAPTER TEN
DIAGNOSTIC TESTS

Although the experienced clinician may be able to produce a 'diagnosis' just by taking a careful history, many clinical decisions depend on the results of tests to help define the diagnosis. These tests may include a physical examination of the patient, a simple test such as urine examination or a more complicated test such as magnetic resonance imaging (MRI) to see the detailed anatomy of the brain, or a coronary angiogram to outline the anatomy of the coronary arteries.

All of these tests, including the history itself, are subject to inaccuracies and we need to ask 'to what extent do they help with making a true diagnosis?'

INACCURACIES IN THE TESTS
....

Variability
The first type of inaccuracy that may be introduced concerns the variability of the actual clinical measurement. Studies have shown that different nurses measure blood pressure differently, different doctors come to different conclusions about the same patients' histories, different radiologists put different interpretations on the same X-ray pictures. Whilst these examples are due to the observer (the nurse or doctor), other differences are caused by variability in the subject (patient) from time to time in measurements such as blood glucose which are related to the body's diurnal rhythms.

Let us take the example of measurement of blood pressure. In a cross-sectional survey in an industrial population,[1] it was found that when five nurses measured blood pressure, the mean systolic pressure varied from an average of 141.5 mm Hg in measures made by Nurse 1, to an average of 132.5 mm Hg in measures made by Nurse 5. This is an example of observer variation and is an important source of systematic bias in the interpretation of blood pressure levels which can be minimised by training the observers. An even greater variation was seen when the blood pressures of the lightest people in the same survey (average, 132.7 mm Hg) were compared with the heaviest (average, 150.0 mm Hg). Blood pressure is measured clinically by inflating and deflating a cuff wrapped around the upper arm. These results reflect the known association between blood pressure and weight, but the authors speculated that some of the apparent effect among the heavy subjects may have been due to the cuff failing to fully encircle the arm. Measures may vary in a random manner, rather than as in the systematic examples given above. As well as the systematic variation with time of day of biological measurements, there is in addition a random element which, whilst not usually leading to bias, does decrease the likelihood of observing a true difference between study groups.

Validity

Validity is defined by Last[2] as 'an expression of the degree to which a measurement measures what it purports to measure'. In the context of diagnostic tests, we try to compare the results of the test with a 'gold standard' or truth concerning whether the condition is present or not. Such a comparison enables us to determine how well the test actually identifies this truth.

Any test may be considered in terms of its validity, and its components are termed sensitivity and specificity. These are derived by considering a table of the general form of Table 10.1. At the top of the table is 'truth', the real answer as to whether the disease is present or absent. Along the side is the positive or negative result of the test used.

Table 10.1 Comparison of diagnostic test with reality.

Result of test	Disease present	Disease absent
Positive	a	b
Negative	c	d
	$a + c$	$b + d$

There were a subjects recorded who genuinely have the disease in question and in whom the test was positive. There were c subjects recorded who also have the disease, but in whom the test was negative. The ability of the test to pick out those people who truly have the disease is called the sensitivity of the test and is calculated as a percentage:

$$\text{sensitivity} = 100 \times a / (a + c)$$

Conversely, the test has correctly identified *d* subjects as not having the disease, but there are *b* subjects labelled positive when in fact they do not have the disease. The ability of the test to say disease is absent when it is truly absent is called the specificity of the test and is calculated as a percentage:

$$\textbf{specificity} = 100 \times d / (b + d)$$

An exercise stress test is often used to help with the diagnosis of ischaemic heart disease (coronary artery disease is another name for the condition where the blood supply to the heart muscle is inadequate for the work it has to do). The 'gold standard' in this case is a coronary angiogram where the anatomy of the coronary arteries can be clearly seen and the degree of obstruction to the blood supply determined. Table 10.2 shows how the stress test performs in comparison with the angiogram—in this table 900 of the 1000 people tested actually have the disease.[3] We find a sensitivity of 71% and a specificity of 73%, as follows.

Table 10.2 Comparison between results of a stress test and a coronary angiogram in the diagnosis of heart disease.

| | *Coronary angiogram* | | |
Exercise stress test	*Disease present*	*Disease absent*	*Total*
Positive	639	27	666
Negative	261	73	334
	900	*100*	*1000*

Sensitivity:
639/900 = 71% (i.e. 71% of those with the disease have a positive test).
Specificity:
73/100 = 73% (i.e. 73% of those without the disease have a negative test).

Reading the figures the other way round, of the 666 people who test positive on the stress test, 639 actually have the disease (96%). This statistic is called the positive predictive value and tells us that in this clinical setting, in which 90% of people have the disease, nearly all of those who test positive actually have the disease. On the other hand, only 73 of the 334 people who test negative really do not have the disease (22%). This statistic is called the negative predictive value and in this example the test is leading the clinician to falsely reassure a large number of people who, even though they have tested negative, actually have the disease in question.

Positive predictive value:
639/666 = 96% (i.e. 96% with a positive test truly have disease).
Negative predictive value:
73/334 = 22% (i.e. 22% with a negative test truly do not have disease).

Table 10.3 presents a quite different scenario where only 200 of the 1000 tested actually have the disease. The sensitivity and specificity are the same as in Table 10.2 but, with the change in prevalence, the positive and negative predictive values have changed markedly. Now the exercise stress test misleads the clinician into falsely worrying people that they have the disease when in fact the angiogram shows that they are disease-free.

Table 10.3 Comparison between results of a stress test and a coronary angiogram in the diagnosis of heart disease—same sensitivity and specificity as in Table 10.2, but lower disease prevalence.

Exercise stress test	Coronary angiogram		
	Disease present	Disease absent	Total
Positive	142	216	358
Negative	58	584	642
	200	800	1000

Positive predictive value:
142/358 = 40% (i.e. 40% with a positive test truly have disease).
Negative predictive value:
584/642 = 91% (i.e. 91% with a negative test truly do not have disease).

The important principle here is that the interpretation of a positive or negative test depends on the frequency (prevalence) of the disease in the population in which the test is being used. It is vital that the clinician assess this in advance in order to be able to interpret the result of the test; another term for this is the pre-test probability.

The other, more complex, issue is whether the test has actually helped, or 'made a difference' to the clinical management of a particular person. If you had reason to believe beforehand that 90 of 100 such people would really have the disease, then an exercise stress test has only increased the probability from 90 to 96 out of 100. If the purpose was to decide if surgery was likely to be helpful or not then you might just as well have gone straight to the angiogram. In fact, a negative result would have been so misleading that it would be truly unhelpful. The test has not 'made a difference'—so why do it?

Note that diagnostic tests are particularly helpful when the pre-test probability is closer to 50% because any change from this is likely to make a difference. A great deal of clinical experience, or access to the appropriate literature, is needed to determine the pre-test probability.

FROM THE CLINICAL TO THE POPULATION SETTING
......

In the usual clinical situation tests are used to help reach a diagnosis in a person who has come to the doctor with a symptom or complaint. The purpose is clearly defined in terms of the particular patient, and the desired end result of the process is to initiate the appropriate treatment. Certain tests are also used widely in community 'screening programmes' of which those aimed at detecting cancer, especially breast or cervical, or cardiovascular disease, are perhaps the best known. Screening is defined as 'the presumptive identification of unrecognised disease or defect by the application of tests, examinations or other procedures which can be applied rapidly. Screening tests sort out apparently well persons who probably have a disease from those who probably do not'.[2] There are differences in this use of tests; the subjects generally feel quite well until told otherwise by the programme organisers; the prevalence of the conditions being sought in a community is quite different from that found in a population of 'patients'; the purpose is not to 'make a diagnosis' but rather to delineate a 'high risk' group; and the tests, of necessity, cannot be as searching as those used in a diagnostic situation. We need to use the same type of thinking about the validity of screening tests, as for diagnostic tests, in order to assess their value when used to screen apparently well communities. In addition, notions of cost and benefit need to come into the equation. Sometimes this presents little difficulty but more usually, especially in the case of cancer, problems abound and these are well illustrated in terms of screening the female population for breast cancer.

Mammography, in which X-rays are used to diagnose breast cancer, is in many ways an ideal screening test. When used on a mass scale the test is not especially expensive, the procedure is rapid and painless, and randomised trials have shown that in women over the age of 50 screening produces a very real reduction in the death rate from this common disease. In 1995 a review of the literature on the efficacy of screening mammography was carried out, with the end point being death from breast cancer during the follow-up period.[4] The authors identified eight randomised controlled trials and, in the age group 50–74, in Figure 10.1 the relative risk of death, comparing the screened group to the unscreened group, is shown for each trial identified by its city of origin (in New York the major trial was carried out by the Health Insurance Program and is known as the HIP trial).

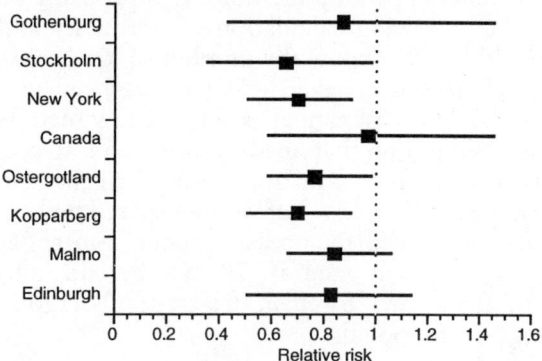

Figure 10.1 *Relative risk of screening mammography in each of eight randomised trials where the end point is death from breast cancer during the follow-up period. The horizontal lines indicate the 95% confidence intervals for the relative risk.*

In such a measure of efficacy a relative risk of 1.00 would show no effect of the screening, a risk of 0.5 would suggest that the risk of dying of breast cancer had been halved, a risk of 2.0 on the other hand would mean a doubling of the risk. In the figure the relative risks are shown and the horizontal lines indicate the 95% confidence intervals for the relative risk. Inevitably there is variation in the relative risk estimates with, in some cases due to relatively small numbers, fairly wide confidence limits. Nevertheless, agreeing with the overall impression of all relative risks being below unity, it is now generally accepted that screening for breast cancer with mammography is a valuable tool in preventive medicine, for women aged 50–74, although reservations are still held by some.

There are two aspects to consider and the first relates to the fact that mammography shares with all other screening tests a risk of misclassifying individuals. Some women are told that they need further investigation for cancer when in fact cancer is absent and, conversely, some are reassured when unfortunately cancer is indeed present. In a recent report from a breast cancer screening programme in Sydney,[5] of the 18 961 women screened 208 were referred for surgical assessment. This assessment, including as it did biopsy, confirmed the presence of cancer in only 105. The positive predictive value of mammography in this region was thus 105/208 or 50.5% which means that almost half the women referred to the surgeons were submitted unnecessarily to a period of acute anxiety, a far from painless procedure, and a dollar cost both indirectly through health insurance schemes and directly in 'topping up' the benefits paid by the fund. It is probably impossible to obtain reliable data allowing calculation of sensitivity and specificity because one would need to know the number of 'true' cancers present in those screened negative, nevertheless it has been estimated that some 10–15% of early breast cancers are missed by mammography.[6]

The second consideration that needs to be taken into account before a screening test is made freely available lies in the balance between the cost in dollars and the gain in lives of women spared by early diagnosis. The results of the Swedish breast cancer controlled trials of mammography[7] for women aged 50–74 may be laid out as in Table 10.4. The data from two Swedish trials in Ostergotland and in Kopparberg have been pooled.

Table 10.4 Pooled results of two Swedish trials of breast cancer mammography in women aged 50–74, up to eight years follow-up. Deaths are from breast cancer.

Group	Population	Observed deaths	Rate per 10 000	Expected deaths	Attributable lives 'saved'
Screened	58 148	71	12.2	108	37
Control	41 104	76	18.5		

If the breast cancer death rate (over eight years) in the control group of women is applied to the group offered screening, then we can calculate the number of deaths that would have been expected in the latter group had they not been screened. This allows for an estimate of the 'attributable risk' of screening; note that in this context the word 'risk' actually describes a benefit.

Presumably as a consequence of the programme and subsequent treatment, we may estimate that 37 women in the screened group had their deaths postponed. To achieve this, the cost at the first level was the screening of 1572 women for each life saved. On the second level, account must be taken of all the indirect costs, such as time lost from work, travel, home care, and the costs of investigating those women who turn out to be 'false positives'. One estimate is that each life 'saved' costs $US1.2 million,[5] but it needs to be realised that such estimates are but rough approximations based on very soft data. In any case, whether such expenditure is 'worth it' is very much a matter of judgement, a judgement dependent on other calls on the national purse at a particular time.

Economists have used two methods, cost benefit analysis and cost effectiveness analysis, to relate costs to benefits. In cost benefit analyses the cost of medical care is balanced against the loss of net earnings due to death or disability. Cost effectiveness analysis compares similar ways of achieving a specified health benefit in terms of the dollar cost of the different strategies or treatments.

Other problems in the evaluation of screening programmes

Early detection of disease in asymptomatic people through screening is gaining increasing favour as a method of improving the health of populations yet the evaluation of such programmes is less simple than might appear. One of the earliest demonstrations of this followed intense mass-radiography campaigns in the United Kingdom—the purpose of which was to lower tuberculosis notification rates. To quote Wilson and Jungner[8] '...Thus in England and Wales (following campaigns) in 1938–39 the mean annual notification rate per 100 000 persons was 88; in 1947–50 it rose to 100 per 100 000, and this was followed by a fall in 1954–55 to 80 per 100 000 persons'. These authors illustrated the situation by a diagram, similar to that reproduced here as Figure 10.2. It is apparent that the tuberculosis notification rates had been falling for a number of years due to improved nutrition, housing and the introduction of effective drug therapy. The effect of the screening programme was to produce a temporary rise in notification rates due to diagnosis of new cases much earlier than would have occured without the programme. Since the underlying incidence of the

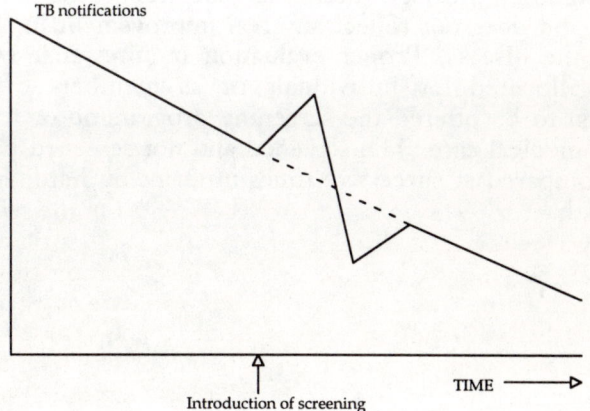

Figure 10.2 *Effect on tuberculosis notifications of a mass radiography screening programme.*[8]

condition had not been changed, apart from the general decline, this rise in rate was succeeded by a compensatory fall and then a return to the original baseline. In such a situation it would be extremely doubtful whether the community received any long-term benefit, in spite of the promoters of the campaign pointing out its apparent case-finding virtues. On the other hand, for an individual to be diagnosed earlier, and to be given effective treatment, could make an enormous difference to that person's life. Throughout the discipline of public health this conflict between what is good for the individual and what is good for the community provides a constant source of tension appearing in many guises and is apparently insoluble in all of them.

Another aspect of the evaluation of screening programmes which can produce erroneous answers is known as 'lead–time bias'. To consider this we will develop an hypothetical situation, illustrated in Figure 10.3. Let us suppose that two women each develop breast cancer at the same time and that eventually each dies of this disease, also at the same calendar time. The first woman (A) has her cancer diagnosed by her doctor whom she consults when she first notices a lump in her breast. The second woman (B) has a screening test for breast cancer and, as a consequence, her cancer is diagnosed much earlier than that of woman A, and she receives appropriate treatment. One way of evaluating the effectiveness of screening is to compare the survival time of patients diagnosed through screening with the survival times of patients diagnosed in the usual manner. Of our two women, the time of survival from diagnosis to death is much longer in the woman whose cancer was diagnosed early by screening than in the woman diagnosed through the usual channels. This difference is artefactual and does not reflect any real improvement in the natural history of the disease. Proper evaluation requires that women are randomly allocated (as individuals or as members of different populations) to be offered the screening programme or to continue with usual medical care. The screened and not screened populations are then compared at successive times in terms of 'hard' end points, such as death.

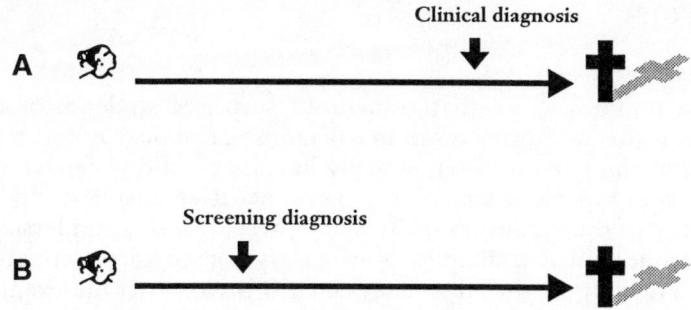

Figure 10.3 *Lead-time bias: a comparison between the fate of two women, one whose breast cancer was diagnosed through usual care and the other by a screening campaign.*

EXERCISES

Exercise 10.1

A man goes to see his doctor because he has been experiencing chest pain. The doctor takes a history and, principally on the basis of this, decides that coronary heart disease (CHD) is a strong possibility because the history is quite typical of angina. The doctor also examines the patient, although this cannot actually help diagnose CHD, because finding other evidence of arterial disease or risk factors, such as high blood pressure, would increase the probability of disease being present. As a consequence, the doctor thinks that an exercise stress test would be appropriate and the result is positive. The next thing to do is a coronary angiogram. Do you think that this patient is closer to the Table 10.2 situation (a pre-test probability of disease of 90%) or to Table 10.3 (20%) and why?

Exercise 10.2

A 55-year-old woman complains to you about the unnecessary anxiety she experienced following a screening mammogram. Although this was reported as 'abnormal' the subsequent biopsy, which was rather painful, showed no cancer. How would you explain to her the benefits of a breast screening cancer programme?

ANSWERS

Exercise 10.1
A piece of knowledge that sometimes surprises students of health sciences is that a positive result in a diagnostic test does not necessarily mean that the person tested actually has the condition for which the test is being performed. Nor does a negative result exclude the possibility of the condition really being present. A clear understanding of epidemiological principles is necessary for correct test interpretation. We suggest that this case scenario is closer to the example in Table 10.2 with a high pre-test probability of 90%.

Exercise 10.2
As in the case of clinical diagnostic tests, knowledge of sensitivity, specificity and predictive values will provide the foundation for an explanation of how a screening test, such as mammography, could 'get the wrong answer'. We also might need to explain why it is generally thought that the benefits to the community, and to individuals, of a mammographic screening programme are greater than the disadvantages including, as they do, an unavoidable number of 'false alarms'.

CHAPTER ELEVEN

RANDOM VARIABLES & DISTRIBUTIONS

INTRODUCTION

The importance of statistical inference in epidemiology, and in medicine in general, follows from the need to extrapolate from samples to populations, from the particular to the general. In a drug trial, for example, we want to extrapolate the trial results to a wider group of people than just those in the trial. In a case-control study of benzene exposure and leukaemia, the outcome is worth reporting because it is applicable to a larger population that those in the study.

The second reason for the central role of statistical inference in epidemiology is that with human data there is always unexplained variation that is large enough to be important. This is due to the inherent complexities of biological and social mechanisms, and shows up in variation in measurements between people, and even on the same people at different times. Epidemiology does not have the luxury of precision that the so-called 'exact' sciences share.

POPULATIONS AND SAMPLES

The relationship between a sample and the population from which it is drawn is crucial to statistical inference. We often want to find out about a characteristic of a population, such as the mean systolic blood pressure of 20-24-year-old women, or the percentage of fibre in the diet of school children, or the relative risk for pancreatic cancer, comparing diabetics with non-diabetics. Such population characteristics are called **parameters**. A large part of the enterprise of epidemiology is concerned with making inferences about parameters: estimating them, comparing parameters in different sub-populations, and so on. But in general this cannot be done by examining the whole population of interest.

Suppose that we are interested in the mean cholesterol level of Australian adult males, or the slope and intercept of the line which relates the expected blood pressure of an individual to their age. It is either not possible or impractical to try to determine the exact value of the quantity of interest. We can obtain an **estimate** based on a sample; with a well designed sample, or study, we can obtain a very good estimate, which will be quite sufficient for practical purposes. The key requirement of the sample or study is that it be designed in such a way that it gives us an unbiased estimate of the population parameter. Much of the earlier chapters have been concerned with methods for good design.

POINT ESTIMATION
....

Usually it is straightforward to obtain from the sample a **point estimate** of the relevant parameter. To estimate the mean blood pressure of the population we would calculate the mean blood pressure of the people in the sample. To estimate the dietary fibre intake of school children we would calculate the sample percentage. A point estimate is useful in giving us a quantitative impression about the parameter.

However, to make a credible inference about a parameter it is necessary to go beyond point estimation, for two reasons.

Intuitively, we know that an estimate from a large sample is better than an estimate from a small sample. Reporting the point estimate alone does not convey this.

Secondly, a variable that takes a large range of values will have its mean estimated less precisely than the mean of a variable which is always in a narrow band. We would be more confident of the precision of our estimate if we estimated the mean weight of newborn babies from a random sample of 100 such babies, than if we estimated the mean weight of adult men from a random sample of 100 adult men, because the weight variation among the babies would be much less than among the men.

The two considerations of sample size and the variation in the variable being measured mean that a point estimate of a parameter is an inadequate basis for a complete inference about the parameter. Point estimates are essential, but they are not enough.

RANDOM EXPERIMENTS

To go beyond point estimates it is necessary to introduce a structure to the population whose parameters we are trying to estimate, and to the sampling procedure we use. We start with the idea of a **random experiment**.

A random experiment is a procedure leading to an observable outcome, with the purpose of obtaining information. So any epidemiological study can be considered a random experiment, whether it is a cohort study, a randomised trial, a case-control study, or a survey: before we carry out the study, we are uncertain about the outcome. The word 'random' is therefore being used here to convey uncertainty, rather than to mean haphazard or chaotic.

A simple example is this: a coin is tossed three times, and the uppermost face is recorded each time.

An epidemiological example is this: a group of 20 patients with carcinoma of the colon is selected and observed, and the times from date of diagnosis until death are noted.

Clearly, in the first example it is easier to list the set of possible outcomes, but even in the second, we could describe beforehand the set of possible outcomes in principle. In both cases, before we make the observations, we are uncertain which of the possible outcomes will eventuate. It is in this sense that we denote that experiment as 'random'.

We assign a probability to each possible outcome. Probability is a number between 0 and 1, which reflects the chance of an outcome occurring. The scale is from 0 to 1, with 0 representing impossibility and 1 certainty, although sometimes the percentage scale is used: 'the chances are 60%', meaning a probability of 0.6.

Probability may be assigned to outcomes in a number of ways. With simple structures like tossing a fair coin, appeal to symmetry may be possible. For the coin-tossing example above, each of the eight possible outcomes: *hhh, hht, hth, thh, tth, tht, htt, ttt,* (where *tht*, for example, means a tail, then a head, then a tail) is equally probable on grounds of symmetry. So each outcome is assigned the same probability, 1/8. Another method of assigning probabilities is to use the long-term limit of the proportion of times an event occurs, in a hypothetical sequence of repetitions of the random experiment.

RANDOM VARIABLES AND PROBABILITY DISTRIBUTIONS
....

A **random variable** is a variable measured in a random experiment. Random variables are denoted by capital letters, usually towards the end of the alphabet.

For the colon cancer example, the following random variables could be defined (as well as many others):

X = number of patients still alive five years from date of diagnosis;
Y = time between date of diagnosis and death for patient no. 7.

There are two distinct types of random variables that we consider:
1. Discrete random variables take only particular (discrete) values and are usually counting variables taking the values 0, 1, 2, ... Of the two above, X is a discrete random variable.
2. Continuous variables can take any value in an interval. Y is a continuous random variable.

Random variables have probability distributions associated with them. For discrete random variables, we can define $\Pr(X = 15)$, which reads as 'the probability that X takes the value 15', $\Pr(X \geq 10)$ and so on.

Consider the coin-tossing example. We could define the random variable Z to be the number of 'heads' obtained. By looking at the outcomes which give the possible values of Z we see that $\Pr(Z=0) = 1/8$, $\Pr(Z=1) = 3/8$, $\Pr(Z=2) = 3/8$ and $\Pr(Z=3) = 1/8$. By referring back to the outcomes which result in particular values for the random variable, we can build up the probability distribution of a random variable.

To specify the probability distribution of X in the colon cancer example, we need to define $\Pr(X=0)$, $\Pr(X=1)$, ... $\Pr(X=20)$. These probabilities must individually lie in the range from 0 to 1, and collectively add up to 1, since they apply to mutually exclusive events which exhaust all the possibilities.

Usually probability distributions are defined by developing a formula for $\Pr(X=x)$. For the colon cancer study, if it were assumed that each patient had a probability, p, of surviving five years, and that the survival prognosis for any single patient was independent of all the others, then the probability distribution of X would be the **binomial distribution**:

$$\Pr(X = x) = \frac{20!}{(20-x)! \; x!} \, p^x(1-p)^{20-x}, \; x = 0, 1, \dots , 20$$

Note that the symbol $n! = n \times (n-1) \times \dots \times 2 \times 1$. For example, $3! = 3 \times 2 \times 1 = 6$. Also, $0! = 1$.

The way in which this distribution is derived is beyond the scope of this text, but it follows the procedure of referring back to the outcomes which result in particular values for the random variable.

Note that this distribution is completely specified except for p, the probability of five-year survival. We have thus arrived at a typical situation, in which a probability distribution for a random variable has been defined, but there is an unknown parameter. The remaining task is to estimate that parameter.

The distribution of X for various values of p, the probability of five-year survival, is shown in Figures 11.1 to 11.3. From Figure 11.1, for example, it can be seen that if $p = 0.1$, the chance that none survive is about 0.12, the chance that 3 out of the 20 survive is just under 0.20, and so on.

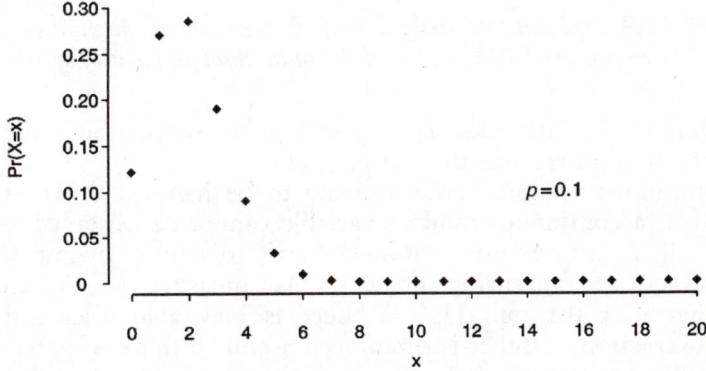

Figure 11.1 *Probability distribution of X, the number surviving 5 years, when 20 patients are followed up and the individual probability of survival is 0.1, or 10%.*

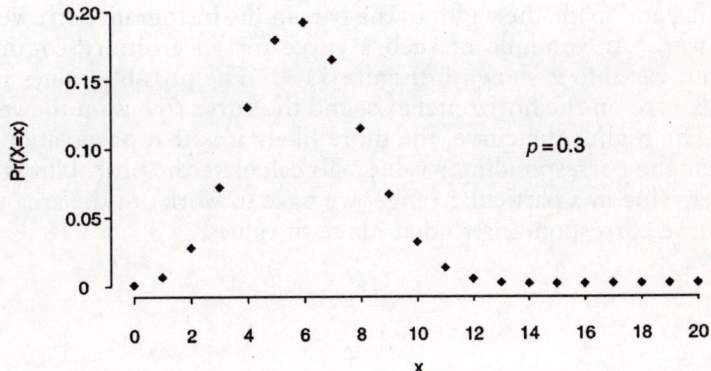

Figure 11.2 *Probability distribution of X, the number surviving 5 years, when 20 patients are followed up and the individual probability of survival is 0.3, or 30%.*

119

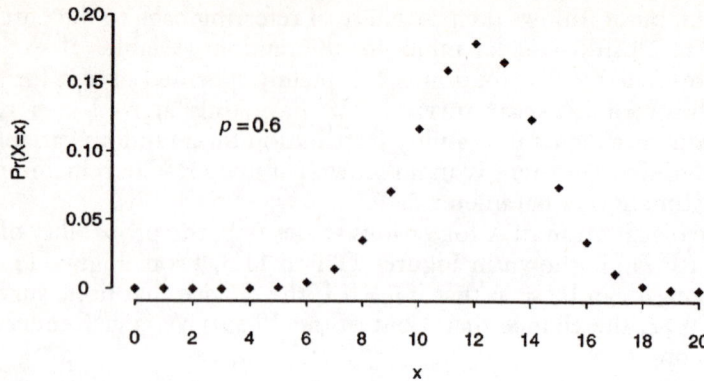

Figure 11.3 *Probability distribution of X, the number surviving 5 years, when 20 patients are followed up and the individual probability of survival is 0.6, or 60%.*

The binomial distribution is only one of many distributions that a discrete random variable may have.

Continuous random variables need to be handled differently. In principle, a continuous random variable cannot be observed exactly, since all measurements are necessarily discrete, owing to the inaccuracy of measuring devices. We measure to the nearest centimetre or 0.1 mm Hg, so there is inevitable discreteness in our observations. But it is often very useful to think of variables as essentially continuous.

A continuous random variable *Y* has its probability distribution described by a curve. This curve can be thought of as the histogram that you would get if you obtained many observations on the random variable, and made the width of the bars in the histogram narrower and narrower. An example of such a curve for an arbitrary continuous random variable is shown in Figure 11.4. The possible values that *Y* can take are on the horizontal axis, and the curve *f(y)* is on the vertical axis. The higher the curve, the more likely it is that observations will be near the corresponding *y* value. To calculate the probability that *Y* takes a value in a particular range, we have to work out the area under the curve corresponding to that range of values.

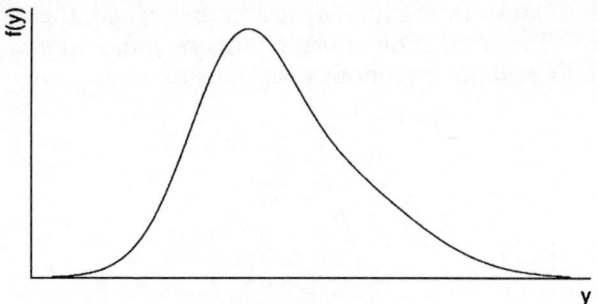

Figure 11.4 *Probability distribution of an arbitrary continuous random variable.*

The most important distribution for continuous random variables is the **normal distribution**, which is symmetric about a central point μ, and bell-shaped. The general normal distribution is shown in Figure 11.5. It is possible to work out probabilities for a normal distribution from statistical tables or software. These probabilities depend only on μ and one other parameter, σ, which specifies the spread of the distribution.

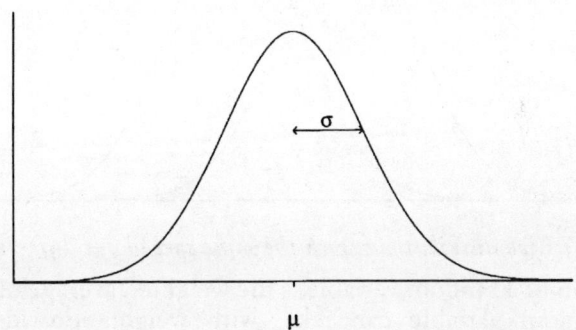

Figure 11.5 *Distribution of a normal random variable.*

MEAN AND VARIANCE

It is laborious to always describe a probability distribution in full. The ideas of **location** and **spread** are fundamental in summarising economically the distribution of random variable. These are illustrated in Figures 11.6 and 11.7; in the first figure, two distributions have the same location but different spread, and in the second, the same spread but different location. The most common and important way to indicate the location of a random variable is to use the **mean**.

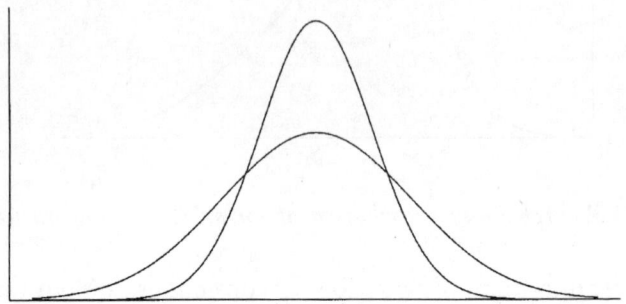

Figure 11.6 *Two distributions with the same location but different spread.*

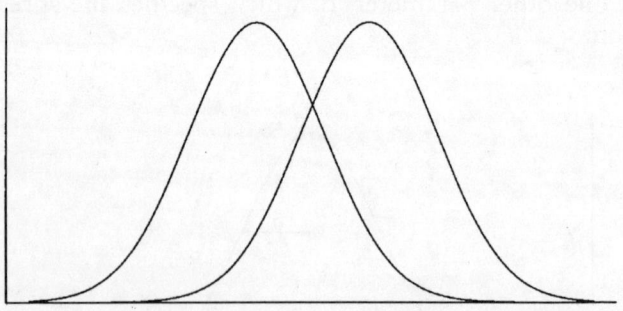

Figure 11.7 *Two distributions with the same spread but different location.*

The mean of a random variable is the weighted average of the values that a random variable can take, with weights provided by the probability distribution. The mean is, in fact, at the centre of mass of the distribution. For this reason, it is at the axis of symmetry for a symmetric distribution. The mean of a binomial random variable is np, and the mean of a normal random variable is μ. The mean is a parameter of the distribution, usually unknown. We are often interested in estimating the mean, and the next chapter discusses this. The mean of a random variable is to be distinguished from a sample mean which can be calculated directly from data.

Knowing the mean of a distribution is useful, but clearly limited, because it needs to be supplemented with information about the spread of the distribution. The most useful measure of spread is the **variance**, which is the weighted average of deviations from the mean, with weights provided by the probability distribution. The more spread out the distribution, the bigger the variance. The variance is especially useful because the variance of a sum (or difference) of independent random variables is equal to the sum of the individual variances. However, the variance is not in the units of the random variable, and the **standard deviation** is defined as the square root of the variance; it is in the units of the random variable. For many distributions, about 95% of the distribution lies within two standard deviations of the mean. The standard deviation of a binomial random variable is $\sqrt{np(1-p)}$, and the standard deviation of a normal random variable is σ.

If a continuous random variable Y has a normal distribution with parameters μ and σ, then the chance that Y is within one standard deviation (σ) of the mean μ is 0.68, or 68%, within two standard deviations, 0.95, or 95%, and within three deviations, 0.997, or 99.7%. We can write the result for two standard deviations like this:

$$\Pr(Y - 2\sigma < \mu < Y + 2\sigma) = 0.95$$

and this is a result which becomes useful in the context of statistical inference, described in the next chapter.

EXERCISES

Exercise 11.1
Which of the following random variables are discrete, and which are continuous?
1. Ten AIDS patients are treated with a new drug; X = the number still alive after one year.
2. A factory is assessed for potentially hazardous pollutants; Y = concentration of trichloroethylene (in mg/m³).
3. Z = the number of female deaths which will occur in Australia in 2005.

Exercise 11.2
A survey of school children in Canberra, in 1990, found that 56% of students aged 13–15 had skin with a detectable level of skin damage due to sun exposure.[1] The students in the study came from nine schools, randomly chosen; within each school two classes were chosen at random.
1. What is the population in this case?
2. Comment on the likely representativeness of the sample.
3. Is the figure of 56% a population parameter, or a sample estimate?
4. What further piece of information would be helpful in assessing the results of the study?

ANSWERS

Exercise 11.1

X and Z are discrete random variables, and Y is a continuous random variable. It might be reasonable to model X as a binomial random variable.

Exercise 11.2

1. The population appears to be school children aged 13–15 living in Canberra in 1990.
2. The sample has elements of random selection. In fact, it is what is called a cluster sample, because the population has been divided into 'clusters' of school classes, and classes, rather than children, have been sampled. This is a convenient strategy, and likely to produce a representative sample, although in general the precision of the study is less than with a simple random sample of the same size.
3. The 56% is a sample figure; it is a point estimate of the true population figure.
4. The extra piece of information is the size of the sample. In fact, there were 'approximately 450' in the sample, and, of these, skin damage data was obtained on 349. It is certainly relevant to ask about the discrepancy between these two figures, and the authors explain the causes and their possible effects on the interpretation of the results.

CHAPTER TWELVE

STATISTICAL INFERENCE

CONFIDENCE INTERVALS

In the section on point estimation in the previous chapter we observed that finding a point estimate of a parameter is useful, but not enough; it does not give any idea of how much that point estimate might be in error. It is helpful to supplement the point estimate with an interval, or range of values, within which we are fairly sure—say with probability 0.95—that the unknown parameter will lie. Such an interval is called a **confidence interval**.

In this section we will derive a confidence interval in a particular context, namely, for a mean of a normal distribution with known variance. It is more important to obtain an appreciation of the meaning of a confidence interval than to understand the technical aspects of this derivation.

Suppose that the serum uric acid level of males (in mg/100 mL) is known to follow a normal distribution with standard deviation $\sigma = 0.9$. A random sample of 100 males is taken, and the observed sample mean level is found to be 5.50. As we saw in Chapter 11, this can be thought of as a point estimate of μ, the population mean. What we are going to do now is to find a confidence interval for μ, around that point estimate of 5.50.

To derive the confidence interval we need a little theory. First, note that the sample mean is a random variable; before we take the sample, we do not know what it will be. The notation we use for the sample mean, considered as a random variable, is $\overline{X}$, whereas the notation we use for the observed value of the sample mean—in this case 5.50—is $\bar{x}$. The idea that $\overline{X}$ can be considered as a random variable with a distribution may seem strange. The way to think about this distribution is to imagine repeated samples of size n, each obtained under the same conditions. The first observed value of the sample mean might be 5.48, the second 5.56, the third 5.49, and so on.

As more and more samples were obtained, the pattern of the distribution of the observed $\bar{x}$s would emerge. In the long run, with an infinite sequence of such samples, we would get the distribution of the random variable $\bar{x}$. So the distinction between $\overline{X}$ and $\bar{x}$ is important; $\overline{X}$ is a random variable with a probability distribution, while $\bar{x}$ is simply a number. In spite of the importance of the distinction, both $\overline{X}$ and $\bar{x}$ are at various times called the sample mean, so it may be necessary to look at the context to see which is meant. The observed value, $\bar{x}$, is an estimate of the population mean μ.

In the example, it is assumed that the serum uric acid level follows a normal distribution, with unknown mean μ (which we wish to estimate) and standard deviation $\sigma = 0.9$. Further, it is assumed that the level in each male is independent of the level in any other. In these circumstances, it turns out that the sample mean, $\overline{X}$, itself follows a normal distribution, with the same mean μ, but with standard deviation equal to $\frac{\sigma}{\sqrt{n}}$, where n is the size of the sample, in this case 100. The derivation of this result is beyond the scope of the text, but it reflects the statements about the accuracy of point estimates in Chapter 11. The standard deviation, $\frac{\sigma}{\sqrt{n}}$ indicates the precision of $\overline{X}$ as a point estimate of μ.

What tends to make $\frac{\sigma}{\sqrt{n}}$ small? Firstly, the smaller σ is, the smaller $\frac{\sigma}{\sqrt{n}}$ is; σ is a measure of the variation in serum uric acid level. This is the effect of 'inherent variation'. Secondly, the larger the sample size, n, the smaller $\frac{\sigma}{\sqrt{n}}$ is: this is the sample size effect. When $\frac{\sigma}{\sqrt{n}}$ is small, the sample mean is a precise estimator of μ.

We can use the distribution of $\overline{X}$ to get a **confidence interval** for μ. Recall that the chance of a normally distributed random variable lying within two standard deviations of its mean is 0.95, so for this particular normally distributed random variable:

$$\Pr(\overline{X} - 2\tfrac{\sigma}{\sqrt{n}} < \mu < \overline{X} + 2\tfrac{\sigma}{\sqrt{n}}) \approx 0.95.$$

In words, this says: the chance that μ lies between the two limits $\overline{X} - 2\frac{\sigma}{\sqrt{n}}$ and $\overline{X} + 2\frac{\sigma}{\sqrt{n}}$ is 0.95, or 95%.

This looks like a probability statement about possible variation in μ, but it is not; μ is a fixed but unknown parameter. It is the interval which is random and the statement says that if many samples of size n were obtained, then for about 95% of these repetitions this random interval would contain the parameter μ. It must be stressed that this sequence of repetitions is imaginary; its purpose is to indicate the interpretation of a particular confidence interval. Figure 12.1 illustrates the situation; the true value of μ, shown in the figure, is unknown in practice. There is a fixed unknown parameter, represented by the vertical solid line, and random intervals which may contain it; in the long run, 95% of the intervals contain the true value, and 5% do not.

(The notation (a, b) is used for an interval, or range, so if we write (2.1, 4.5) we mean all values between 2.1 and 4.5 inclusive.)

Thus the interval $(\bar{x} - 2\frac{\sigma}{\sqrt{n}}, \ \bar{x} + 2\frac{\sigma}{\sqrt{n}})$ is called a 95% confidence interval for µ.

In the example, the observed $\bar{x}$ was 5.50, and n was 100. So the 95% confidence interval for µ is $(5.50 - 2 \times \frac{0.9}{10}, \ 5.50 + 2 \times \frac{0.9}{10})$, ie (5.32, 5.68).

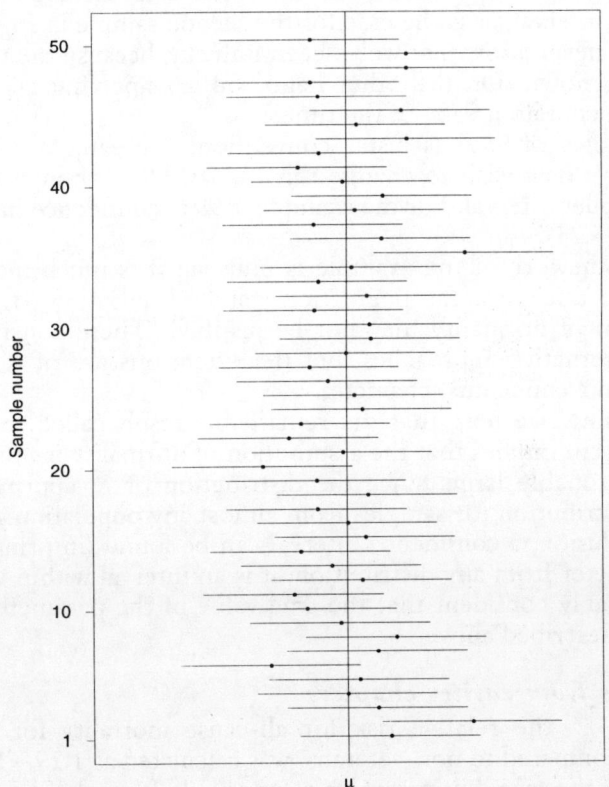

Figure 12.1 *Hypothetical repetition of 50 samples, showing the point estimates, which are the observed sample means (solid dots), the 95% confidence intervals around the estimates (horizontal lines) and the true value of µ.*

In the case of the example, we might say that we are '95% sure that μ lies between 5.32 and 5.68'. What this means is that if we had many such samples, and we calculated the confidence interval in the same way each time, 95% of the intervals would contain the true value of μ. One in every twenty intervals will not contain the true value—μ is not a random variable; it is just a number. In any particular confidence interval, including the one we have just calculated, μ either is or is not in the interval, though we do not know which.

In practice, we do not obtain many samples under the same conditions. So we may happen to be unlucky, in the sense that our sample may be one of the cases in which μ is excluded from the calculated interval, as is the case for the second sample in Figure 12.1. Again, we never know that we've been unlucky, because the true value of μ is unknown. On the other hand, we are applying a procedure which will contain μ 95% of the time.

The choice of 95% is just a convention; if greater confidence is required we may wish to change this to, say, 99%, though the price paid is a wider interval. For the example, a 99% confidence interval for μ is (5.27, 5.73).

The framework of the example is unusual; it is much more likely that we do not know the population standard deviation (σ), and the assumption of normality may not be justified. These considerations lead to alternative approaches, but the extensions are of a technical rather than a conceptual character.

(In passing, we note that the remarkable result called the central limit theorem implies that the assumption of normality is unnecessary if n is reasonably large, since the distribution of $\overline{X}$ approximates a normal distribution for samples from almost any population.)

In conclusion, a confidence interval can be found (in principle) for any parameter from any distribution; it is an interval within which we are reasonably confident that the true value of the parameter lies, in the sense described above.

Examples from earlier chapters

In Table 5.2, the relative risk for all-cause mortality for Vietnam veterans, compared to non-veterans, was calculated as 1.29. This is an estimate of the true, but unknown relative risk. It can be shown that a 95% confidence interval for the relative risk is (1.09, 1.53).

In the survey cited in Table 6.1, 81/364, or 22.3% of women agreed or strongly agreed with the statement: 'There is really no way I can solve the problems I have'. This result from the survey was an estimate of the true percentage of women in that category, in the source population. A 95% confidence interval for the true percentage is (18.0, 26.5).

Table 7.5, concerned with mortality in Victorian doctors, actually presents confidence intervals. Note the effect of sample size in that table: the SMR for male doctors, based on 115 deaths, was 0.59, with a 95% confidence interval of (0.49, 0.71). There were only 11 deaths among the much smaller female doctor population, which gave an SMR of 0.84, and a 95% confidence interval of (0.42, 1.51); quite a bit wider than for the males. For a rare outcome, with very few observations, the confidence interval is even wider: the SMR for suicide among the female doctors was 5.01, but this was based on only 3 observed deaths (and 0.6 expected), and the 95% confidence interval is consequently very wide indeed: (1.03, 14.7).

Confidence intervals are a very helpful and economical way of expressing the precision of an estimate, and research journals in the medical field urge authors to present their key results in this way.

HYPOTHESIS TESTING
·······

The formulation, testing and refining of theories form a major part of epidemiology. We may wish to test whether a new drug is more effective than the previously best available, or to test a theory that a new therapy regime will prolong the lives of cancer patients, or to investigate the possibility of an association between a certain feature of lifestyle and the incidence of coronary heart disease.

We shall consider the whole concept of hypothesis testing in the context of the colon cancer example (see Chapter 11). In the example, we have previously considered the random variable X = number of patients still alive five years from the date of diagnosis, and we assumed that:

$$\Pr(X = x) = \frac{20!}{(20-x)! \, x!} \, p^x (1-p)^{20-x}, \; x = 0, 1, \dots , 20$$

where p is the probability of five-year survival for an individual patient.

Suppose it were 'known' that, in general, the five-year survival rates for colon cancer patients were 30%. (In fact, in England and Wales for persons first diagnosed in 1975 the five-year relative survival rates were 31% for men and 30% for women.) Before advancing further with this example, it should be pointed out that it is being used to illustrate statistical principles only, and in practice the assumptions made and methods used would be different; a randomised controlled trial would be an appropriate study design.

The 20 patients we are considering have been subjected to a new chemotherapeutic programme. Does this regime improve their survival? This question could be answered in the terms of the statistical theory of hypothesis testing. The idea is to quantify the weight of evidence in favour of the treatment.

There are some extremes worth considering. Firstly, note that if this group of 20 is like other patients, the mean number of survivors is $(20\times0.3) = 6$: on average, about six will survive at least five years. The actual distribution of patients surviving is binomial with $n = 20$ and $p = 0.3$. We have already seen this distribution plotted, in Figure 11.2, and for convenience it is repeated here, as Figure 12.2. We can see from the distribution that (when $p=0.3$) the probability of observing 12 or more is very small.

If all 20 survived, therefore, we would be confident that the survival rate was higher on the new regime, and it would be tested more thoroughly on larger numbers of patients. On the other hand, if six survived, this would suggest that the new treatment had done nothing in particular, since we would expect about six on known rates. Finally, if none survived, we would conclude that the treatment was ineffective; in fact, we would question whether it had had a harmful effect, since Figure 12.2 shows that (when $p = 0.3$) the probability of observing zero (out of 20) is also very small.

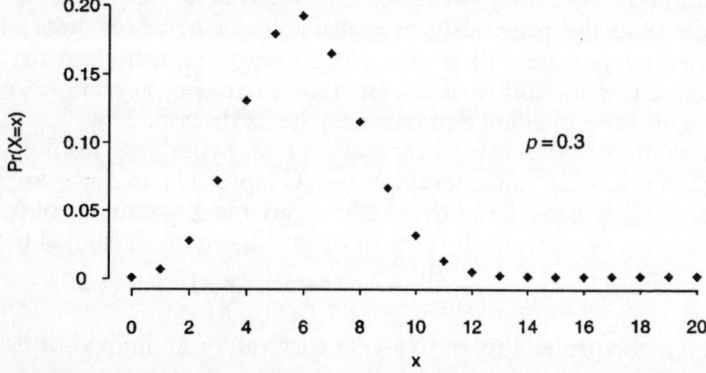

Figure 12.2 *Probability distribution for the number of colon cancer survivors, when the probability of 5-year survival is $p=0.3$.*

Between 6 and 20 is a grey area. What if 9, or 11, survived? Clearly such results would be in favour of the treatment, but would they be convincingly so?

We now frame this problem as an hypothesis test. A statistical hypothesis is a statement about some population. In the example, the distribution of the random variable X is completely specified except for the probability of survival, p. We are interested in whether the survival rate of the 20 is the same as usual, or better. Expressed mathematically, we wish to test the hypothesis that $p = 0.30$ against the alternative that

$p > 0.30$. The first of these hypotheses would be called the null hypothesis, and is usually denoted by H_0. It often represents the status quo, reflecting the weight of established evidence. Usually, we are attempting to 'refute' the null hypothesis; of course, we are not doing that in a logico-deductive sense, but by the weight of empirical evidence.

The alternative hypothesis—in this case $p > 0.30$—is denoted by H_1. The null and alternative hypotheses are the only two considered, so with the problem as it stands we are excluding the possibility of the treatment programme making things worse, that is, $p < 0.30$.

In some hypothesis testing contexts, one may actually have to make a choice, in practical terms, between the two hypotheses, after the data are collected. For example, the physicians running the study may decide that if the observed value of X is at least 10, they will regard this, for practical purposes, as evidence that H_1 is true. That means that in the grey area between 6 and 20 (referred to above), they have settled on a threshold, or critical value of 10. Nine or fewer surviving does not convince them that H_0 is false; ten or more surviving does convince them: they will reject H_0 and favour H_1. Because H_0 and H_1 are hypotheses, they will never really know if they have made the right decision. But it is possible to define and control two types of errors that they could have made. The situation is as shown in Table 12.1.

Table 12.1 Possible outcomes when testing an hypothesis.

	Decision	
Actual situation	*Do not reject H_0*	*Reject H_0*
H_0 *True*	Correct decision (probability $1-\alpha$)	Type I error (probability α)
H_1 *True*	Type II error (probability β)	Correct decision (probability $1-\beta$)

A **type I error** is rejecting the null hypothesis when it is true. The probability of a type I error is called the **level of significance** of the test, and is denoted by the Greek letter alpha (α). In the example, to work out α we need to calculate the probability that X is at least 10, given that $p = 0.3$.

This probability turns out to be 0.05, using the formula for the binomial distribution (this can also be seen, approximately, from Figure 12.2). So the investigators have accepted a risk of 0.05—a chance of 1 in 20—of rejecting H_0 when it is true, that is, of saying there has been a real improvement in survival ($p > 0.3$) when, in fact, there has been no improvement ($p = 0.3$).

A **type II error** is made when the null hypothesis is not rejected, but H_1 is true. The probability of a type II error is commonly denoted by the Greek letter beta (β).

We would like both α and β to be small, so that we are making correct decisions most of the time. But there is a trade-off here; if we make α too small, not only do we tend to avoid rejecting H_0 when it is true (a good thing), we also make it unlikely that we will reject H_0 when it is false, and H_1 is true (a bad thing). Thus by decreasing α we increase β, and some compromise is necessary—we cannot make α as small as we please. Historically, the values of α most widely used have been 0.05 (1 in 20) and 0.01 (1 in 100).

The **power** of the test is the probability of rejecting H_0 when H_1 is true; clearly, we would like this to be large. The power is equal to $1-\beta$. The type I and type II errors are described in the context of a drug trial in Chapter 13.

Note that in determining α for a given test, or determining the test for a given α, the distribution of some statistic, assuming that H_0 is true, must be known. These distributions are not always straightforward, and so information corresponding to $\alpha = 0.05$ and 0.01 is tabulated. However, with the advent of computers and readily available statistical packages, the complexity of the distributions is less of a problem.[1] This makes possible the use of an alternative, more informative, approach to hypothesis testing. The **P-value** is defined as follows:

P= Pr (result at least as extreme as that obtained, given that H_0 is true).

Very roughly, the P-value answers the question: 'What are the chances of getting this result, assuming H_0 is true?'

Here 'extreme' is determined by the alternative hypothesis. (P is the standard notation for the P-value. It should not be confused here with p = probability of five-year survival.)

Suppose that, at the end of the colon cancer study, eight patients survived. On the basis of the investigators' rule, we do not reject H_0, since the observed X is less than 10. We might say that 'the results were not significant at the 5% level'; the 5% here refers to the probability of a type I error, 0.05.

Using a P-value approach, we would calculate the chance that X is greater than or equal to 8, assuming that H_0 is true. This probability is found to be 0.23. We might say that 'the P-value was 0.23'.

The P-value indicates how unlikely the observed sample is, assuming that H_0 is true. A very small P-value indicates that if H_0 is true, something very unlikely has occurred. This causes us to question the premise, H_0. One can think of the argument as a probabilistic version of *reductio ad absurdum*; we assume H_0 (the premise) and then show that the chance of obtaining our actual results is very small (and analogous to a contradiction in the *reductio ad absurdum* reasoning). Therefore, we doubt H_0 (analogous to proving the premise is false). By quoting the P-value we impart more insight than the simple conclusion to reject or not reject the null hypothesis. In the example, whether $X = 10, 11, \ldots, 20$ we reject H_0, but these outcomes represent degrees of decisiveness concerning the evidence. This is reflected in the P-values corresponding to these outcomes, shown in Table 12.2.

Table 12.2 P-values for hypothetical outcomes in the colon cancer example.

observed X	7	8	9	10	11	12	13	... 20
P-value	0.39	0.23	0.11	0.05	0.02	0.01	0.00	0.00

The P-value, then, indicates the strength of evidence against H_0; the smaller the P-value, the stronger the evidence against the null hypothesis. The P-value cannot be interpreted as the chance that the null hypothesis is true. It is calculated assuming that the null hypothesis is true.

A bonus of the P-value approach is that it diverts attention away from the often artificial accept/reject alternative. By merely quoting a P-value, we leave it to the experimenter to make any appropriate decision.

We have seen that the power of the test, $1 - \beta$, is the probability of rejecting H_0 when H_1 is true, and that it is desirable for the power to be large. In the example, what is the power when $p = 0.5$? It is equal to Pr (reject H_0, given that $p = 0.5$) = Pr $(X \geq 10$, given that $p = 0.5) = 0.59$; we obtain this probability by looking at the binomial distribution with $n = 20$ and $p = 0.5$.

Note that the power depends on the particular value of the parameter under consideration. Further, in the example the power is not very great; there is only just a better than even chance that we will pick up a true improvement in survival rate from 0.3 to 0.5. This is due to the small numbers of patients.

In the example, the alternative hypothesis, H_1, is one-sided: $p > 0.3$. However, a two-sided alternative could have been taken: $p \neq 0.3$. Whether one chooses a one- or two-sided H_1, depends on one's beliefs before the study. In the context of the example, choosing a two-sided alternative would imply the *a priori* belief that the treatment might improve or **make worse** the survival rate. On the other hand, choosing a one-sided alternative would imply the belief that the therapy could be beneficial, but could not be harmful.

If a particular one-sided alternative hypothesis is true, the corresponding one-sided test is more powerful than the two-sided test, but to use a one-sided test we must be certain that we can exclude some values of the parameter altogether. It is often the case that we do not have any *prima facie* reason to exclude some values, and in this event the widest possible alternative—two-sided—is called for.

If the test is two-sided, the P-value is defined to be twice the P-value of the relevant one-sided test. Thus, in the example, when we observed eight patients dying, for a two-sided test, $P = 2 \times 0.23 = 0.46$.

In this chapter, two methods of making inferences about a parameter were presented: confidence intervals and hypothesis tests. Which is better? They have a complementary relationship; a confidence interval consists of those values of a parameter which would not be rejected by an hypothesis test. If the 95% confidence interval includes the null value, then $P > 0.05$, and if it does not, then $P < 0.05$. A confidence interval is more informative than an hypothesis test; it implicitly performs hypothesis tests for all possible H_0 values of the parameter, and gives a range within which we are reasonably sure the parameter lies.[2,3] Hypothesis tests are useful if the problem is exclusively concerned with testing a claim.

The reader is referred to standard texts for more detailed discussions of estimation and hypothesis testing.[4-6]

EXERCISES

Exercise 12.1
Consider Figure 12.1 again, the diagram illustrating the concept of confidence intervals.
1. How many of the 50 intervals contain the true value, μ? Does the answer surprise you?
2. If you had obtained one of the samples for which the 95% confidence interval did not contain μ (e.g., sample 2), what could be done about that?
3. If the sample size was increased from 100 to 1 000 for all of the samples in the hypothetical repetition, would a greater proportion of the 95% confidence intervals contain μ? Explain.

Exercise 12.2

When opinion polls are published in a major Australian newspaper, they are often supplemented with the information that 'for a sample of this size, the maximum likely error is about 3%'. The sample size for this statement is 1 000. Put this statement within the framework of confidence intervals.

Exercise 12.3

In a study of liver cancer in Aboriginal Australians,[7] the authors reported that the relative risk of primary hepatocellular carcinoma (PHC) in the Northern Territory, comparing Aboriginals with non-Aboriginals, was 10.4, with a 95% confidence interval of (4.0, 26.6). In conjunction with the confidence interval, they reported a *P*-value: $P < 0.001$.

1. What is the parameter being estimated?
2. Could the true value of the relative risk be 1? 20? 100?
3. What is the null hypothesis being tested?
4. What is the meaning of the *P*-value in this case?
5. The authors reported a 95% confidence interval. Would a 90% confidence interval be narrower, or wider?
6. Would a 99% confidence interval include 1? What about a 99.9% confidence interval? Give reasons.

ANSWERS

Exercise 12.1

1. 48 out of the 50 intervals contain the true value, and 2 do not; the true value, μ, is below the lower limit of two of the intervals (samples 2 and 35). 48/50 is 96%, not 95%; but the 95% is a long-term average, not (necessarily) the percentage which will cover the true value in any actual sequence. In fact, the number of intervals, out of 50, which will cover the true value, is a binomial random variable with $n = 50$ and $p = 0.95$.
2. You could do nothing at all about it, for the simple reason that, in practice, you do not know the true value of μ, so you are not aware that you have obtained a confidence interval which does not include it. You simply report the confidence interval, and it has the same status as any other reported interval.
3. If the sample size is increased, the percentage covering the true value does not change; the percentage is determined by the '95%'. What will happen, however, is that the confidence intervals will become narrower.

Exercise 12.2

This statement is essentially about a confidence interval: with a random sample of size 1 000, the 95% confidence interval for any percentage has width (at worst) 6%, that is ±3%. So, for example, if the survey has found that the Prime Minister's approval rating is 43%, a 95% confidence interval for the true approval rating is (40%, 46%). Near election time, this possibility of sampling error is particularly relevant; if one is estimating a percentage close to 50%, the error of ±3% can mean the difference between a poll being 'correct' and 'incorrect'.

Exercise 12.3

1. The parameter being estimated is, in some sense, the 'general' relative risk for PHC, comparing Aboriginals to non-Aboriginals. The population studied was the Northern Territory, between 1980 and 1989. One can imagine an extrapolation in both time and space: in other areas of Australia, and for other periods of time, including, potentially, the future. Without such extrapolation, statistical inference is not really an issue; we simply have a numerical fact.

2. The true relative risk could be any of these values. But the confidence interval only includes one of them—20—and it is this one with which the data are more consistent. As measured by the 95% confidence interval, the data are not consistent with a true relative risk of 1 or 100, because it excludes both these values.

3. The null hypothesis is that the true relative risk is 1; this is the natural hypothesis of 'no effect', or no association between the factor (race) and the outcome (PHC).

4. The P-value was very small: $P < 0.001$. This means that the chance of observing a relative risk as large as that obtained (i.e. 10.4) is less than one in 1 000, if there is genuinely no association between PHC and Aboriginality.

5. A 90% confidence interval would be narrower than the 95% confidence interval. The lower (higher) the level of confidence, the narrower (wider) the confidence interval.

6. If the 95% confidence interval includes the null hypothesis value, then the P-value is larger than 0.05, and if it does not, then the P-value is smaller than 0.05. There is a similar correspondence for other values. In the example, $P < 0.001$, so both the 99% and 99.9% confidence intervals would not include the null hypothesis value, 1.

CHAPTER THIRTEEN

SAMPLE SIZE

Problems with sample size, or 'how many subjects (or animals) do you need?', are an important part of the planning of most forms of medical research. In statistical terms, the larger the study, the more powerful the hypothesis test and the narrower the confidence interval. What this means in practice is that a study of inadequate size may miss something important that would have been detected in a larger study. We have already touched on this point in the colon cancer example in Chapter 12, in which the null hypothesis that the five-year survival rate, p, was 0.3 was tested against the alternative $p > 0.3$. With a study group of size 20, and level of significance $\alpha = 0.05$, the power for $p = 0.5$ was only 0.59. In Table 13.1, the power for various sample sizes and values of p are given.

Table 13.1 Power for various values of the sample size n and survival rate p, for testing $H_0: p = 0.3$ against $H_1: p > 0.3$ with $\alpha = 0.05$ (see colon cancer example, Chapter 12).

	n, sample size		
p, survival rate	20	50	100
0.33	0.09	0.12	0.12
0.35	0.12	0.19	0.23
0.40	0.24	0.44	0.62
0.50	0.59	0.90	0.99

The table shows that to have a test with power = 0.90 for finding a true increase in five-year survival rate from 0.3 to 0.5, 50 subjects are needed. The effect of increasing the sample size can be seen; this would be regarded as quite an acceptable level of power, in contrast to the power of 0.59 for a sample of size 20. If the sample size was 100, the power would be even larger. If the smallest true effect that we want to detect is very large, a small study will suffice, because a dramatically large effect will tend to show itself quite obviously in the results. On the other hand, if the effect of practical interest is quite small, we are going to need a very large study, to detect it with high probability. Many studies have inadequate statistical power,[1] and medical journals now urge authors to present a power-based assessment of study size in submitted articles.

The effect of increased sample size may be expressed in another way. The *P*-value in the example was 0.23, indicating that nothing very unusual had happened, if H_0 were true, and implying no special reason to doubt H_0. This was from a sample five-year survival rate of 8/20 = 0.40.

Suppose, however, that the **same** sample survival rate had been observed in a larger study. What, then, would be the *P*-value? Table 13.2 addresses this question.

Table 13.2 *P*-value for testing H_0: $p = 0.30$ against H_1: $p > 0.30$, for various values of the sample size *n*, when the sample survival rate is 0.40.

	n, sample size					
	20	**30**	**40**	**50**	**100**	**200**
No. surviving 5 years	8	12	16	20	40	80
5-year survival rate	0.40	0.40	0.40	0.40	0.40	0.40
P-value	0.23	0.16	0.12	0.08	0.02	0.002

The interpretation of this is that, if H_0 is true, a sample survival rate of 0.40, above the expected value of 0.30, is not particularly surprising in a sample of only 20 subjects. But it is quite unusual if it comes from a sample using 100 subjects, and it is remarkable if the sample is 200 subjects, even though in each case the point estimate—0.40—is the same.

RANDOMISED TRIALS

For the rest of the chapter we will be referring to sample sizes required for randomised controlled clinical trials, but the same principles apply to other research designs.

In the simplest kind of drug trial we take a group of patients with the condition in question and randomly allocate them to two groups—one to receive drug A and the other to receive drug B (or placebo). We then proceed and see which treatment is better. How many patients do we need?

Firstly, recall that in the conclusions of the study there are two kinds of errors that can be made; either may be dangerous under certain circumstances.

Type I: Rejection of the null hypothesis when it is true. The null hypothesis in this context is 'Drug A has the same effect, on average, as drug B'. A type I error is committed when the conclusion is that drug A is better (or worse) than drug B, when it really is not. If the study results had favoured drug A, this might result in a lot of people being put on drug A which may be much more expensive than drug B and may have more serious side effects.

Type II: Accepting the null hypothesis when it is false. The conclusion is that drug A and drug B are no different when (e.g.) really drug A is a lot better. This could result in a lot of people being deprived of a good treatment.

No matter how well a study is designed, one of these errors may be made, but they may be made unlikely by appropriate choice of sample size.

There are three questions to consider at the outset.

1. How big a risk are we willing to run so that, when the experiment is over, we conclude that the two treatments **are** importantly different, when in fact they are not? This risk is simply the probability of a type I error, so the question may be rephrased as 'What level of significance will be used in the test?' Traditionally $\alpha = 0.05$ is used. It is important to understand that the value of α is unavoidably arbitrary, but $\alpha = 0.05$ is the typical value.

2. Suppose that there really is a difference between the two treatments, how big must this difference be before it is important not to miss it? The answer to this question comes out of clinical experience and common sense. Factors that must be taken into account include the seriousness of the condition; age-group; and the cost, painfulness and side-effects of the new treatment. For example, one might well think a 5% difference in treatments for childhood leukaemia is worthwhile detecting, whereas a 20% difference in treatment for headache might need to be present before one would recommend a change from simple, cheap and reasonably safe aspirin. We, therefore, need to specify the 'important difference', that is the minimum difference we wish to detect.

3. If there really is an important difference, what should the chances of detecting it be? This is the power of the test, that is the probability of picking up a difference that is really there. Many investigators use a 90% level; if there really is a difference (of specified magnitude) then they want to be 90% sure of detecting it.

COMPARING TWO PERCENTAGES
·······

Many clinical trials have dichotomous end-points, 'healed, not healed', 'dead, alive', and so forth. The following discussion deals with such outcomes; different results are available for an outcome which is a continuous variable (such as haemoglobin or cholesterol levels, blood pressure). For dichotomous outcomes the quantity we measure is the percentage of subjects with the outcome of interest. For example, we may be interested in the percentage that survive a given length of time after treatment, or the percentage that show a particular response.

Table 13.3 shows the sample sizes required in each of two equal sized groups, for testing the difference between two percentages.[2] If the null hypothesis is not true, and there is a difference in the percentages of some sort, it is assumed that the first population has the lower percentage and the second population the higher. The body of the table shows the sample sizes. The table assumes that a two-sided alternative hypothesis will be used, that the risk of a type I error, α, is set at 0.05, and that the power is 0.90.

Table 13.3: Sample sizes required in each of two equal-sized groups, for the comparison of two percentages: $\alpha = 0.05$, power = 0.90; percentage in the second population is assumed to be higher than in the first.

%, Popn. 1									

%, Popn. 1	5%	10%	15%	20%	25%	30%	35%	40%	45%
50%	1667	402	171	91	54	34	22	14	6
55%	1633	389	163	85	49	30	18	9	
60%	1564	367	151	77	43	25	12		
65%	1461	337	135	66	35	17			
70%	1323	298	115	53	24				
75%	1151	249	91	36					
80%	944	192	60						
85%	701	122							
90%	420								

Difference between the two percentages (column header spanning 5% through 45%)

Consider the boxed figure of 298 in Table 13.3. This says that if the true percentages in the two populations are 70% and 80%, 298 subjects will be needed in each group, to detect the difference with probability 0.90. So a total sample size of about 600 is needed. The two populations could be all patients given drug A, and all patients given drug B, in terms of the clinical trial discussed above. Or they could be those with the disease and those without the disease, in the context of a case-control study. But it is important to understand that the percentages referred to in the table are the true, unknown percentages in the populations (if the alternative hypothesis is true), not the results in the study itself.

The table illustrates that if we want to detect a small difference, large sample sizes are needed; if the percentage in the first population is 50% and the percentage in the second population is 55%, a total study size of about 3 300 is required.

An argument based on symmetry allows us to use the table for small percentages too; for example, if the two (true) percentages under the alternative hypothesis are 20% (= 100% − 80%) and 30% (= 100% − 70%) then the sample size required in each group is also 298.

Sample size formulae for a wide range of epidemiological study designs are given in Breslow and Day.[3]

EXERCISES

Exercise 13.1

The medical director of a large industrial chemical complex was asked to examine the possibility of a link between exposure to a particular solvent used in one of the plants, and the development of the blood disorder leukaemia.

She decided that a case-control design was appropriate and wrote up a protocol for carrying out the study. This protocol included the proposed study size.

In due course the parent company in the USA approved the project but added the proviso (insisted on by its statistical division) that the study size should be such that the power of the study should be 90%, for a relative risk of 3 and level of significance 0.05. Back home, the Union Health and Safety Committee (after seeking its own advice) was adamant that the power should be 95% for a relative risk of 1.5 and level of significance 0.05.

1. Which proposal (the parent company's or the Union Committee's) gives a larger required study size?
2. Why did the two parties hold such different and strong views on what appear to be mere statistical niceties?

Exercise 13.2

A randomised controlled trial is proposed to study the long-term survival of coronary bypass surgery patients, comparing two different surgical procedures. The investigators want to be able to detect a small benefit: if procedure A is more effective than procedure B, they are interested in designing a study to detect this with high probability, specifically, if the 10-year survival rate for procedure A is 0.90, compared to the expected survival rate of 0.80 for procedure B patients. If they can recruit subjects at the rate of 15 per month, about how long will the recruitment phase need to be?

Exercise 13.3

A researcher comes to you, knowing that sample size is an important issue to address. He says, confidently, that he wants a large enough sample size 'so that at the end of the study, there will be a significant result'. What is your response?

Exercise 13.4

Regarding the size of a study, Miettinen wrote that: 'On the first, and pivotal level the decision is a binary one (the choice between zero and non-zero as the size').[4] What did he mean?

ANSWERS

Exercise 13.1

1. The Union's proposal will lead to a larger study, for two reasons: it regards the smallest effect to detect as being 1.5, which is smaller than the analogous value for the parent company's proposal; secondly, the Union wants a higher statistical power than the parent company.
2. In this situation the Union might argue for the detection of the smallest possible relative risk, with the highest possible power. It would be in the interests of its members to do so. Note that, in practical terms, there is often an intrinsic limitation on the study size; for a rare disorder like leukaemia, studied in a relatively narrow context, cases will be very infrequent. In these situations it may be more useful to turn the calculation around, and determine the power for the given sample size.

Exercise 13.2

From Table 13.3, we see that 192 subjects are needed in each group, or a total study size of about 400. At a frequency of 15 patients per month, that implies a recruitment period of just over two years. In practice, a longer period may be needed, if the rate of 15 patients per month is just the actual rate in the clinics of the study, since one needs to allow for those patients who decline to consent to participate, or are ineligible.

Exercise 13.3

Unfortunately, it is not possible to guarantee a significant result. It is not even possible to make this very likely, in general. If the null hypothesis is actually true, then the chance of a significant result is the pre-set value of α, typically, 0.05. The power only comes into play if the null hypothesis is not true; then we can make sure that the chance of a significant result is high, for a specified alternative hypothesis.

Exercise 13.4

Miettinen was making the point that sample size is only one aspect of study design, and it could be said that it is a somewhat secondary issue. If a study is bound to be biased, because it has a flawed design, then, in a sense, the larger the sample size the worse the situation, since the biased result will be estimated with greater precision.

REFERENCES

Chapter One

1. Christie D, Spencer L, Sentilselvan A (1990). *Respiratory health in the Newcastle area, 1979–1988.* University of Newcastle, Newcastle.
2. NSW Department of Health (1994). Health indicators for NSW 1993. *Public Health* 5: 1–78.
3. Case RAM, Lea AJ (1955). Mustard gas poisoning, chronic bronchitis, and lung cancer. *Brit. J. Prev. Soc. Med.* 9: 62–7.
4. Armstrong BK, de Klerk NH, Musk AW, Hobbs MST (1988). Mortality in miners and millers of crocidolite in Western Australia. *Brit. J. Indust. Med.* 45: 5–13.

Chapter Two

1. Bennett S, Donovan J, Stevenson C, Wright P (1994). *Mortality surveillance, Australia 1981–1992.* Australian Institute of Health and Welfare, AGPS, Canberra.
2. McKeown T, Lowe CR (1974). *An introduction to social medicine.* 2nd ed. Blackwell, Oxford.
3. Australian Institute of Health and Welfare (1994). *Australia's Health 1994.* AGPS, Canberra.
4. Leitch F, O'Connor S, Heller R (1987). Variation in death certification of ischaemic heart disease in Australia and New Zealand. *Aust. NZ J. Med* 17: 309–315.

Chapter Three

1. Britt H, Miles D, Bridges-Webb C, Neary S, Charles J, Traynor V (1993). A comparison of country and metropolitan general practice. *Med. J. Aust.* 159: Suppl.
2. Australian Institute of Health and Welfare (1994). *Australia's Health 1994.* AGPS, Canberra.
3. Alexander HM, et al. (1990). *Risk factor prevalence study 1988–1989 data book.* Hunter Region Heart Disease Prevention Programme, CCEB.
4. Commonwealth Department of Health (1985). *Advancing Australia's Health: draft plan.* AGPS, Canberra.
5. Nutbeam D, et al. (1993). *Goals and targets for Australia's health in the year 2000 and beyond.* Department of Public Health, University of Sydney.
6. Australian Bureau of Statistics (1981). *Causes of Death, Australia 1981.*
7. Australian Bureau of Statistics (1992). *Causes of Death, Australia 1992.*
8. Australian Bureau of Statistics (1992). *Deaths NSW 1992.*
9. Epidemiology and Health Services Evaluation Branch, NSW Health Department (1993). *Health Indicators for NSW 1993.*

Chapter Four

1. Bennett S, Donovan J, Stevenson C, Wright P (1994). *Mortality surveillance, Australia 1981–1992.* Australian Institute of Health and Welfare, AGPS, Canberra.

2. Christie D, Robinson K, Gordon I, Rockett I (1984). 'Health Watch': the Australian petroleum industry health study surveillance programme. *Med. J. Aust.* 141: 331–334.
3. University of Newcastle & NSW Central Cancer Registry (1994). The NSW coal industry cancer surveillance program. Report to the Joint Coal Board, Discipline of Environmental and Occupational Health.
4. Lynch P, Oelman BJ (1981). Mortality from coronary heart disease in the British Army compared with the civil population. *Brit. Med. J.* 283: 405–407.

Chapter Five

1. Doll R, Morgan LG, Speizer FE (1970). Cancers of the lung and nasal sinuses in nickel workers. *Brit. J. Cancer* 24: 623–632.
2. Adena MA, Cobbin DM, Fett MJ, et al. (1985). Mortality among Vietnam veterans compared with non-veterans and the Australian population. *Med. J. Aust.* 143:541–544.
3. Hammond EC, Selikoff IJ, Siedman H (1979). Asbestos exposure, cigarette smoking and death rates. *Ann. NY Acad. Sci.* 330: 473–490.
4. Rose G (1985). Sick individuals and sick populations. *Int. J. Epidemiol.* 14: 32–38.
5. Bradford Hill A (1965). The environment and disease: association or causation? *Proc. Roy. Soc. Med.* 58: 295–300.
6. Rose G (1992). *The strategy of preventive medicine.* OUP, Oxford.
7. Alexander HM, et al. (1990). *Risk factor prevalence study 1988–89* data book. Hunter Region Heart Disease Prevention Programme. CCEB, Newcastle.
8. Intersalt cooperative research group (1988). Intersalt: an international study of electrolyte excretion and blood pressure. *Brit. Med. J.* 297: 319–328.
9. Heller RF, Chinn S, Tunstall Pedoe HD, Rose G (1984). How well can we predict coronary heart disease? Findings in the United Kingdom Heart Disease Prevention Project. *Brit. Med. J.* 288: 1409–1411.
10. Doll R, Bradford Hill A (1966). Mortality of British doctors in relation to smoking observations on coronary thrombosis. National Cancer Institute Monograph 19, W. Haenzel (ed.).

Chapter Six

1. Last JM (ed.) (1983). *A Dictionary of Epidemiology.* OUP, New York.
2. Freud S (1913). *The interpretation of dreams.* (trans. A.A.Brill). George Allen & Unwin, London.
3. Miettinen OS (1985). *Theoretical Epidemiology.* Wiley Medical, New York.
4. Sanson-Fisher R, Schofield M, Mia See (1992). Availability of cigarettes to minors. *Aust. J. Publ. Hlth.* 16: 354–359.
5. Alexander HM, et al. (1990). *Risk factor prevalence study 1988–1989* data book. Hunter Region Heart Disease Prevention Programme, CCEB.
6. Waters WE (1971). Migraine: intelligence, social class and familial prevalence. *Brit. Med. J.* ii: 77–81.
7. Wintrobe MM, Thorn GW, Adams RD, Braunwaid E, Isselbacher KJ, Petersdorf RG (1974). *Harrison's Principles of Internal Medicine.* 7th ed. McGraw-Hill, New York, p. 1865.
8. Christie D, Gordon I, Robinson K, Santamaria J (1986). Unpublished data.
9. Christie D, McPherson L, Kincaid-Smith P (1976). Analgesics and the kidney: a community-based study. *Med. J. Aust.* 2: 527–529.

10. Christie D, Rockett I, et al. (1982). Health Watch: Annual Report 1981. University of Melbourne, Melbourne.

Chapter Seven

1. Case RAM (1958). Mortality from cancer of the lung in England and Wales. In *Carcinoma of the Lung*. J Bignall (ed.), E & S Livingstone, Edinburgh & London.
2. Lancaster HO (1951). Deafness as an epidemic disease in Australia. *Brit. Med. J.* ii:1429–1432.
3. Christie D, Gordon I, Robinson K (1986). Smoking in an industrial population: an analysis by birth cohort. *Med. J. Aust.* 145: 11–14.
4. Christie D (1978). 'The analgesic abuse syndrome': an epidemiological perspective. *Int. J. Epidemiol.* 7: 139–143.
5. Shigematsu I, Kagan A (1986). Cancer in atomic bomb survivors. Gann Monograph on Cancer Research No. 32. Japan Scientific Societies Press, Tokyo & Plenum Press, New York & London.
6. Lilienfeld AM (1976). *Foundations of Epidemiology*. OUP, New York.
7. Christie D, Robinson K, Gordon I, Bisby J (1991). A prospective study in the Australian petroleum industry. I Mortality. *Brit. J. Industrial Med.* 48: 507–510.
8. Vano K, Rhoads GG, Kagan A (1977). Coffee, alcohol and risk of coronary heart disease among Japanese men living in Hawaii. *N. Eng. J. Med.* 297: 405–409.
9. Schlicht S, Gordon I, Ball J, Christie D (1990). Suicide and related deaths in Victorian doctors. *Med. J. Aust.* 153: 518–521.
10. Newcastle Discipline of Environmental & Occupational Health, University of Newcastle & NSW Central Cancer Registry (1994). The NSW coal industry cancer surveillance program.
11. Simonato L, Fletcher AC, Cherrie JW, et al. (1987). The International Agency for Research on Cancer historical cohort study of SMF production workers in seven European countries: extension of the follow-up. *Annals of Occupational Hygiene* 31: 603–623.

Chapter Eight

1. Rothman KJ (1986). *Modern Epidemiology*. Little, Brown and Company, Boston & Toronto.
2. Ross J, Woodward A (1994). Risk factors for injury during basic military training. *J. Occ. Med.* 36: 1120–1126.
3. Cleland L (1987). 'RSI': a model of social iatrogenesis. *Med. J. Aust.* 147: 236–239.
4. Batey RG, Burns T, Benson RJ, Byth K (1992). Alcohol consumption and the risk of cirrhosis. *Med. J. Aust.* 156: 413–416.

Chapter Nine

1. Report to the MRC on their conference on diabetes and pregnancy (1955). The use of hormones in the management of pregnancy in diabetics. *Lancet* ii: 833–836.
2. Herbst A, Ulfelder H, Poskanzer D (1971). Adenocarcinoma of the vagina: association of maternal stilbestrol therapy with tumour appearance in young women. *N. Eng. J. Med.* 284: 878–881.
3. Beral V, Colwell L (1980). Randomised trial of high doses of stilbestrol and ethisterone in pregnancy: long-term follow-up of mothers. *Brit. Med. J.* 281: 1098–1101.

4. Sorenson G, Lando H, Pechacekt T (1993). Promoting smoking cessation at the workplace: results of a randomised controlled intervention study. *J. Occ. Med.* 35: 121–126.
5. Miao LL (1977). Gastric freezing: an example of the evaluation of medical therapy by randomised clinical trials, in *Costs, risks, and benefits of surgery.* Bunker J, Barnes B, Mosteller F (eds.). OUP, New York.
6. Ruffin J, Grizzle J, Hightower N, et al. (1969). A co-operative double blind evaluation of gastric 'freezing' in the treatment of duodenal ulcer. *N. Eng. J. Med.* 281: 16–19.
7. Solomon P, Wilson S, Swanson C, Cooper D (1990). Effect of Zydovudine on survival of patients with AIDS in Australia. *Med. J. Aust.* 115: 254–257.
8. Sidtis J, Gatsonis G, Price W, et al. (1993). Zidovudine treatment of the AIDS dementia complex: results of a placebo-controlled trial. *Ann. Neurol.* 33: 343–349.
9. Ioannidis J, Cappelleri J, Lau J, et al. (1995). Early or deferred Zidovudine therapy in HIV-infected patients without an AIDS-defining illness. *Ann. Int. Med.* 122: 856–866.
10. Jennings C, Barraclough BM, Moss JR (1978). Have the Samaritans lowered the suicide rate? A controlled study. *Psych. Med.* 8: 413–422.
11. The Coronary Drug Project Research Group (1980). Influence of adherence to treatment and response of cholesterol on mortality in the Coronary Drug Project. *N. Eng. J. Med.* 303: 1038–1041.
12. Wilcox RG, Roland JM, Banks DC, et al. (1980). Randomised trial comparing propanolol with atenolol in immediate treatment of suspected myocardial infarction. *Brit. Med. J.* 280: 885–888.
13. Pocock SJ (1983). *Clinical Trials: a practical approach.* John Wiley & Sons, Chichester.
14. Elwood PC, Wood MM (1966). Effect of oral iron on the symptoms of anaemia. *Brit. J. Prev. Soc. Med.* 20: 172–175.
15. Garraway WM, Akhtar AJ, Hockey L, Prescott RJ (1980). Management of acute stroke in the elderly: follow-up of a controlled trial. *Brit. Med. J.* 281: 827–829.
16. Mather HG, Morgan DC, Pearson NG, et al. (1976). Myocardial infarction: a comparison between home and hospital care for patients. *Brit. Med. J.* i: 925–929.
17. Pond S, Lewis-Driver D, Williams G, Green A, Stevenson N (1995). Gastric emptying in acute overdose: a prospective randomised trial. *Med. J. Aust.* 163: 345–349.
18. Whyte IM, Buckley NA (1995). Progress in clinical toxicology: from case reports to toxicoepidemiology. *Med. J. Aust.* 163: 340–341.
19. Conine T, Daeschel D, Hershler C (1993). Pressure sore prophylaxis in elderly patients using slab foam or customised contoured foam wheelchair cushions. *Occ. Therapy J. Research* 13: 101–114.

Chapter Ten

1. Heller RF, Rose G, Tunstall Pedoe HD, Christie DGS (1978). Blood pressure measurement in the United Kingdom Heart Disease Prevention Project. *J. Epidemiol. & Comm. Hlth* 32: 235–238.
2. Last JM (1983). *A Dictionary of Epidemiology.* OUP, New York.

3. Heller RF, Whelan G (1991). Using the diagnostic test. *Med. J. Aust.* 154: 33–37.
4. Kerlikowske MD, Grady D, Rubin SM, Sandrock C, Ernster VL (1995). Efficacy of screening mammography. A meta-analysis. *JAMA* 273: 149–154.
5. Harrison R, Glenn D, Niesche F, Patrick W, Ramsey-Stuart G, Renwick S, Rickard M, West R (1994). Surgical treatment of breast cancer: experience of the Central Sydney Area Health Service breast X-Ray programme 1988–91. *Med. J. Aust.* 160: 617–620.
6. Wright CJ, Mueller CB (1995). Screening mammography and public health policy: the need for perspective. *Lancet* 346: 29–32.
7. Tabar L, Fagerberg C, Gad A, Baldetorp L, Holmberg LH, et al. (1985). Reduction in mortality from breast cancer after mass screening with mammography. *Lancet* i: 829–832.
8. Wilson J, Jungner G (1968). Principles and practice of screening for disease. *Public Health Paper* 34, WHO, Geneva.

Chapter Eleven

1. Fritschi L and Green A (1995). Sun damage in teenagers' skin. *Aust. J. Publ. Hlth* 19: 383–386.

Chapter Twelve

1. Gordon I (1985). Misconception concerning the ubiquitous *P*-value. (Letter). *J. Occ. Med.* 27: 403.
2. Berry G (1986). Statistical significance and confidence intervals. *Med. J. Aust.* 144: 618–619.
3. Gardner MJ and Altman DG (1986). Confidence intervals rather than *P* values: estimation rather than hypothesis testing. *Brit. Med. J.* 292: 746–750.
4. Altman DG (1991). *Practical Statistics for Medical Research*. Chapman and Hall, London 152–178.
5. Armitage P and Berry G (1994). *Statistical Methods in Medical Research* (3rd ed.). Blackwell Scientific, Oxford 93–105.
6. Bland M (1995). *An Introduction to Medical Statistics* (2nd ed.) OUP, Oxford 119–123, 133–147.
7. Wan X, Mathews JD (1994). Primary hepatocellular carcinoma in Aboriginal Australians. *Aust. J. Public Health* 18: 286–290.

Chapter Thirteen

1. Hall JC (1982). The other side of statistical significance: a review of type II errors in the Australian medical literature. *Aust. NZ J. Med.* 12: 7–9.
2. Dobson AJ and Gebski VJ (1986). Sample sizes for comparing two independent proportions using the continuity-corrected arc sine transformation. *Statistician* 35: 51–53.
3. Breslow NE and Day NE (1987). *Statistical Methods in Cancer Research*, vol. 2: *The Design and Analysis of Cohort Studies*. IARC, Lyon.
4. Miettinen OS (1987). *Theoretical Epidemiology: Principles of Occurrence Research in Medicine*. Wiley, New York 62.

INDEX